ᵀᴴᴱ BEST FRIENDS'
GUIDE TO GETTING FIT

D1056703

THE BEST FRIENDS' GUIDE TO GETTING FIT

Kim Murphy
and
Kris Carpenter

Robin,
Read... Enjoy...
Reflect... and
perhaps begin or
reshape your fitness
journey! Kris 2005

Robin ~
wishing you all
the best in your
efforts to get fit
and live well,
Kim 2005

CAPITAL
BOOKS, INC.
Sterling, Virginia

Copyright © 2005 by Kim Murphy and Kris Carpenter

All rights reserved. No part of this book may be reproduced or utilized in any form or by any means, electronic or mechanical, including photocopying, recording, or by any information storage and retrieval system, without permission in writing from the publisher. Inquiries should be addressed to:

Capital Books, Inc.
P.O. Box 605
Herndon, Virginia 20172-0605
www.capital-books.com

Book design and composition by Susan Mark
Coghill Composition Company
Richmond, Virginia

Quotations on pages 14 and 15 from *SIMPLE ABUNDANCE* by Sarah Ban Breathnach. Copyright © 1995 by Sarah Ban Breathnach. By permission of Warner Books, Inc.

ISBN 1-933102-00-4 (alk.paper)

Library of Congress Cataloging-in-Publication Data

Murphy, Kim.
   The best friends' guide to getting fit / Kim Murphy and Kris Carpenter.
      p.   cm.
   Includes bibliographical references and index.
   ISBN 1-933102-00-4 (pbk. : alk. paper)
      1. Physical fitness for women.   2. Female friendship.   I. Carpenter, Kris.
   II. Title.
   RA778.M965   2005
   613.7'045—dc22

                                                2004026314

Printed in the United States of America on acid-free paper that meets the American National Standards Institute Z39-48 Standard.

First Edition

10 9 8 7 6 5 4 3 2 1

Acknowledgments

OUR SINCERE THANKS, to our husbands, Harry and Scott. Thanks seems like such a small word. After all, without you two we never would have met seventeen years ago and been in a position to develop our friendship. Thanks for all the years of love, encouragement, friendship, partnership, and fun that have led up to this point. Thanks too for supporting us as we go way beyond our comfort levels to share such personal and revealing aspects of *all* of our lives. Thanks for being there with us in Virginia Beach and for pampering us, standing beside us, and celebrating with us. It was such a life-changing event that it wouldn't have been the same or half as much fun without you there to share it. And finally, thanks most of all, for being willing to let us fly while still being there to provide the loving foundation we need to stay firmly grounded.

To our boys, Justin, Jason, and Scotty. Thanks for always sharing your enthusiasm, your questions, your encouragement, your ideas, your love, and your faith.

To Don Brazelton. When we first ventured forth on our fitness journey, we had no idea where we were headed. We also had no idea we'd meet someone like you who would be so instrumental in helping us to transform our lives. Thanks for sharing your gregarious, fun-loving, energetic spirit. Thanks for the gentle teasings as you watched us walk or cycle endless, sweatless miles. Thanks for inviting us to your classes and for welcoming us when we eventually joined in. You, better than anyone, know how far we've come. Thanks for leading us there. Most of all, thanks for believing in us, for motivating us, for teaching us how to work through it, how to leave it on the floor, how to unleash the power within our own minds and our bodies. Our hope is that by telling our stories we can indirectly share all that we've learned from you and inspire others in their own fitness journeys.

Contents

INTRODUCTION

On August 31, 2003, we stood at the base of the boardwalk in Virginia Beach, on a warm overcast day, with our arms around each other, beaming with pride. We'd done it. We'd run 13.1 miles—a half marathon. It was the culmination of months, perhaps even years, of dreams, aspirations, discipline, dedication, and hard work. Rather than feeling exhausted, we felt energized, excited, strong, confident, accomplished, and motivated. We were mentally strong, physically fit. We were ready for our next challenge. We had a "bring it on" attitude. It was a feeling of invincibility. One that hasn't dissipated even today.

That's not who we'd always been or how we'd always felt. Few who saw us that day would have guessed that only a few years earlier, we couldn't walk up a gradual hill without getting winded. But it was true.

Yet here we were, at a completely different place in our lives, where exercise was as important to our days as that first cup of coffee. And treating ourselves to daily doses of our friendship while we exercised, was akin to having cream or sugar in our coffee—in other words, you just wouldn't have a cup without it! Amazingly, we had arrived at a place where we knew, finally and without reservation, we had a formula for success—for achieving physical, mental, and spiritual strength.

Without knowing our beginnings—where we started—it would be hard for anyone to really understand the magnitude of our accomplishment,

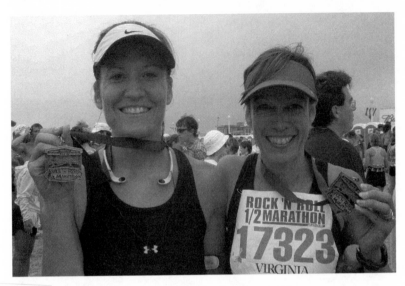

Kris (left) and Kim after Virginia Beach marathon, 2003

of why it meant so much, of all that it represented. Perhaps only the two of us could truly appreciate that. And we both knew full well that we wouldn't have been able to stand there together on that boardwalk, were it not for one another.

Ours is a story of struggles and triumphs—from overcoming devastating health-related battles to combating inner battles of body image and self-control. It's a story of no longer allowing past histories and failures to shape the future. It's a story of friendship and of transformation. It's a story of two different people, with different backgrounds, inclinations, and experiences, arriving at a place together because of each other.

It seemed a story worth telling. Not simply because it involved a success story. That's only a part of it. It seemed a story worth telling because we arrived at a formula for success—one that you, or anyone, can adopt in order to become mentally strong, physically fit.

And if you're reading these pages, we suspect you are searching for that or for something close to it. You may have a list of struggles that you are facing. Some will be similar to ours. Some will be different. You may feel tired. Overwhelmed. Overweight. Unhealthy. Stressed. Exhausted. Drained. Squishy. Listless. Frustrated. Alone. Lost. Weak. Impatient. Frumpy. Stiff. Or, just plain old. Or, perhaps, it's subtler than that. Perhaps you just want to sleep more soundly or wish you had some moments to yourself or you long to feel more light-hearted and uplifted.

Whatever it is you are feeling, let's just agree you're probably not feeling too *fit* right about now.

∽ But What Does That Really Mean? ∽ To Be "Fit"?

According to the President's Council on Physical Fitness and Sports, fitness can be defined as "the ability to perform tasks vigorously and alertly, with energy left over for enjoying leisure time activities and meeting emergency demands. It is the ability to endure, to bear up, to withstand stress, to carry on in circumstances where an unfit person could not continue, and is a major basis for good health and well being."

Attributes of a person's physical fitness level can be measured in a variety of ways, including blood pressure, heart rate, cholesterol level, body fat percentage, weight, and body mass index (BMI). And years of studies have shown that regular exercise can help a person to improve or lower their results in all these areas.

We've come to believe that to be fit speaks about more than just your physical fitness level (the concrete measurements) or whether you can run a mile or two. To be fit is to *feel balanced* in terms of your physical being, your mental state, and deep within your soul. Being fit occurs when all three of these components are in sync and empowered to help you become the best you can be.

It's when your body, your mind, your soul fit together seamlessly, effortlessly, powerfully.

When you become fit, you can transform your life.

Why are we so sure?

Because we've experienced it. We're living it. And if we can live it, you can too. Before we plunge ahead and outline how you can get started on a similar path, let's back up and share our backgrounds with you, so that you can get a better sense of where we started.

∽ "It's Just Stress, Dear"– ∽ Kris Looks Back

As a young child, I always enjoyed physical activity. I biked and played kick ball or volleyball at the neighborhood playground. At the age of seven, I began gymnastics and dance classes. I became obsessed with gymnastics and it became a springboard to my cheerleading career. I cheered for the youth leagues, in high school, and also coached younger cheerleaders. Cheering kept me active and fit.

During my early childhood and high school years I never really considered my eating or exercising habits. I ate what I wanted. Any exercise I did was because I enjoyed the activity. I had a reasonable figure, though it was not necessarily the "ideal" Barbie figure.

When I first went off to college as a freshman, all of the activities that I had been engaged in for so many years stopped. It was the first time I was in charge of managing my own time. Prior to that point, my days were scheduled with practices, dance, and gymnastic classes. Without structured activities on my schedule, I began to experience some weight gain for the first time. Without much thought or a plan, I responded by turning to exercise to improve my appearance. I began to do aerobics with the girls on my dormitory floor. Jane Fonda led us in an hour of kicks, jumps, and grapevines. This little bit of exercise was enough to halt any further weight gain, though it didn't do much to help me shed the weight I'd gained. In order to lose some of that, I began to run. By the end of my freshmen year I trimmed down, but only for a brief time.

As I rolled into my sophomore year and continued on to my senior year, I yo-yoed in terms of weight. Any time I gained more than ten pounds, I would start a jogging routine. That was my primary approach to managing my weight gain. I simply turned to exercise for a while each time I gained weight, but I never stayed the course. I was reactive rather than proactive in my use of exercise.

Upon graduating from college, I became a working girl and spent the greater part of my day behind a desk crunching numbers. Again, I began to put on weight. Again, I used exercise as a quick fix for losing weight, but my demanding schedule meant I was even more sporadic and inconsistent. Exercise was never a priority in and of itself. (It would take years for me to finally discover that exercise could do far more than merely help me manage my weight.)

The long hours at work began to pay off and I was beginning to feel I could ease up a bit on my schedule. I also met my future husband. We were together all the time. He too logged many hours at work, but in his free time he was active. So I followed suit. Prior to meeting him, I had only run or participated in dance or aerobics. He opened up a whole new world of activities to me. Skiing, mountain biking, and softball games became a part of our life together. He was patient in teaching me each new activity and I enjoyed the change. By being in love, not eating much, plus exercising a ton, I lost a lot of weight.

By the time we married, I was very thin. A year into our marriage I became crazy busy with work. My job involved training staff at remote locations, and therefore, weekly travel. Initially, I loved the travel. Since my very first plane trip had not been until I was in college, I was not a worldly individual. Yet here I was, every week, traveling somewhere new: Chicago, Sacramento, Los Angeles, Houston, or Orlando. Not only was it very exciting, it was an awesome opportunity. Again, as work became a greater priority, I made less and less time for any physical activity.

That schedule continued for three to four years and I became exhausted. I vividly remember one trip to Dallas. I had taken an early morning direct flight from Dulles. On it I drifted in and out of sleep. It was not a restful sleep. Once we landed, I collected my luggage. As I did, I realized I was dripping wet. The mere physical activity of collecting my luggage and carrying it through the airport had caused me to sweat profusely. At the time, I remember being very disappointed in myself. I vowed that I would start exercising again to improve my health. I never considered that it was odd for a thin, twenty-six-year-old female to have a racing heart and to be dripping wet in sweat after so little activity. Instead, I attributed it to the hectic pace of my days.

All the professionals and loved ones in my life also attributed the demise of my health to my inability to handle a stressful workload. I was under the care of a doctor because my husband and I were trying to start our family without much success, and even my Ob-Gyn told me that I needed to slow down and be patient.

After a year of trying to conceive, he finally recommended that I have laparoscopic surgery in an effort to find out what was going on.

The procedure revealed that I had one damaged fallopian tube. However, other than that, he said there wasn't any other compelling reason why I had not yet become pregnant. Ironically, after the surgery, I remember the nurses commenting on how fast my heart rate was. They attributed it to my fear and anxiety over the surgery. (Instead, it was a clear sign that there were serious medical conditions going unnoticed.) I continued to feel bad. Worse, I continued to attribute everything to my stressful job. So did everyone else. Then, on one business trip, I visited Houston where my brother and his wife lived. At the time, my mother was also visiting. One night, we were all sitting around having dinner. Then, for no apparent reason I started to have a meltdown. I became extremely angry and began to cry uncontrollably.

This type of behavior had become a frequent occurrence with my husband as well.

It wasn't just my emotions that were off kilter. During one downhill ski trip with my husband and friends, I literally could not catch my breath. At the time I was only twenty-eight years old. My husband looked at me and said, "What has happened to you? You need to start exercising!" It was the first time in my life that I remember not being able to do something physical, relatively easily.

The combination of erratic emotions and failing health, continued to take its toll. My husband and family began to whisper to one another that I needed to consider a career change. They had decided that I was simply not capable of "handling" my stressful job. While I felt the work was challenging, I never thought that it was too much to handle. If anything, my career was clicking along at a great pace.

As the months wore on, I continued to spiral out of control. I was having trouble figuring out how to fix it—and me. As in the past, I turned to exercise. Only this time, things were different. I started to try to run to get back into shape. But I found it impossible. When I ran I could barely catch my breath. I was stunned and decided I no longer liked physical activity. So, I started to avoid it altogether. More time passed. I became an emotional and physical wreck and finally bought into the notion that I simply could not handle the workload. I was starting to believe I was heading for a breakdown.

Finally, my stepmom noticed that my goiter looked extremely enlarged. She suggested that I consult a different doctor. Thankfully, I sought the help of an endocrinologist. He diagnosed me with Grave's disease. I had an overactive thyroid.

The treatment involved destroying half of my thyroid through an oral dose of radioactive iodine. Finally, I began to feel better. Actually I felt better than I had felt in years, despite the fact that I gained twenty pounds.

Once again, I began to run. This time my body cooperated. Quickly, I established an exercise routine—again my sole method of combating weight gain. After losing ten of the twenty pounds, I finally became pregnant. It seemed I was back on track.

I was thrilled to become a new mom. With a new baby, life changed dramatically. There no longer seemed to be any time to exercise—once again exercise slipped down the priority queue. Still, I was content with my body. A year after my son was born we began to hope for another child.

This would be the start of a long, torturous time. For six years, from the ages of thirty-two to thirty-eight, I would endure more medical procedures and disappointments than in all my years leading up to that point. It was marked by endless rounds of medical tests, heartbreaks, pelvic pain, questions, surgeries, false hopes, a devastating miscarriage of twins just days before September 11, and the final realization that perhaps I had become too old to continue to try to conceive. Although it was a physically difficult and emotionally draining six years for me, it marked the start of my journey toward wellness and *true* fitness. It's where the real story begins.

∾ Sizes 6 to 16, and Everything ∾ in Between Kim Looks Back

When I was nine years old, my best friend, Laurie, was playing at my house. She put on a pair of my shorts, pulled them up to her waist, buttoned them, and let go. Stunned, I watched them slide to her knees. It was the very first time I remember realizing that people's bodies were different from one another's. Compared to her, I suddenly felt huge (though I had never felt large at any point until then).

As a kid, I was active but never athletic. I rode my bike, played hopscotch and foursquare, and spent hours twirling on the metal bars until the backs of my knees were a deep crimson. But during recess, when it came time to pick teams for kick ball, I was always one of the last kids picked. I came to hate the idea of sports and dreaded anything related to gym class.

At thirteen, I visited my grandparents and met one of my second cousins. She was quite a bit older than me. She had a lovely face, but was overweight. After she left, my grandmother turned to me and said, "Be careful, or someday you are going to be just like Lili." I was appalled. I couldn't imagine being as big as Lili. And I certainly couldn't imagine what my grandmother saw in me to make her think I'd turn out that way.

But she was a wise soul.

Within a few years of that remark, I had embarked on what would become a lifelong struggle with my weight and body image. By my senior year in high school, I was trying all of the most popular weight-loss methods—from Slim-Fast to Dexatrim to Weight Watchers—with varying degrees of success. I always succeeded at losing, although never at keeping the weight off.

For my mother, my weight problems and lack of activity were maddening, because she was highly disciplined in her eating and exercising—whether she was running, playing tennis, or gardening.

"You need to go out and exercise," she would say, not realizing that I had absolutely no clue as to where to even begin.

When I went away to college, the dieting cycle worsened. I didn't stop at gaining the traditional "Freshman Fifteen," instead going for the record-breaking "Freshman Fifty." In fact, I gained so much weight, so quickly, that even today it's difficult for me to look at pictures from that time.

One summer, I ate only every other day. Imagine that, eating only every other day. I was also a heavy smoker, consuming close to two packs of cigarettes a day (even more on my nonfood days.) Such behavior caused me to swing wildly from one size to another.

In the spring of my junior year, I set out on yet another diet. This time, while everyone else went on spring break, I stayed at school and starved myself. I didn't eat for nearly a week, surviving on cigarettes and Diet Cokes. After I was convinced that my "stomach had shrunk," I lived on Lean Cuisines and salads. It worked (for a time) and I lost a substantial amount of weight.

By the time I headed home that summer, I was smaller than I had been in a long time. I also started exercising for the first time in my life.

Every morning I awoke and did aerobics. Living mostly on beer, popcorn, Diet Cokes, and cigarettes, I plummeted to my all-time low of 107 pounds. I was in heaven (but clearly, had a warped view of what heaven should be). I did enjoy the exercising, but most of all, loved getting dressed without worrying about how I looked in an outfit—because at 107, everything looked pretty darn good. I entered a whirlwind summer romance and all seemed right with the world. Until I returned to school.

Returning for my senior year meant another round of changes. Gone were my morning workouts. Gone was my summer romance. Back came the eating and, shortly thereafter, the weight. And then some. Once again, I outdid myself and gained more weight than ever before, racing from 107 to 178 pounds—in only nine months. By graduation, I had outgrown my size 16 clothes, but wouldn't dare buy a larger size.

After graduation, I went to work, settling into a nine-to-five schedule. For the most part, being in a stable routine helped stop my drastic cycles of extreme dieting. However, by then the damage to my body as a result of all the abusive treatment was extensive. After years of vacillating between starving and binge eating, my metabolism was shot. It didn't know whether to burn calories or to hoard them for fear that future food would be scarce. During one vacation marked by frequent restaurant meals, I gained ten pounds in a single week.

Over the next several years, my weight stabilized a bit. I met the man who would become my husband and we started our family. We had two sons, twenty-one months apart and I worked part-time from home as a freelance writer.

On the one hand, I felt incredibly blessed. We were succeeding at building the kind of home and family life that we both wanted. On the other hand, I was often overwhelmed by the challenges of mothering two active toddlers, trying to run a freelance business, and managing a household.

Because I was always busy, I didn't eat regular meals. Instead I nibbled the boys' Mac and cheese leftovers and snacked throughout the day. I was thinner than I'd been in years, yet I was no longer consciously trying to lose weight. Ironically, that scared me to death. Since I had always gained weight so easily, I figured something was horribly wrong. I couldn't possibly become thin without working at it.

So I went to the doctor for a checkup.

She proclaimed me healthy and sent me on my way.

Perhaps my weight was at an acceptable level, but I felt tired, stressed, and emotionally drained. That spring my husband came home on Mother's Day with a beautiful exotic potted orchid. As I placed it in the center of the dining room table I started to sob. How in the world was I going to cope with having one more living thing that needed me to care for and nurture it?

Clearly, I was far from "healthy." By July the orchid was dead.

∽ From Meltdowns to Marathons ∽

As you can tell from our backgrounds, while the details may vary, we're really not all that different from you or from your girlfriends or from women you meet every day. This is our story—a story of how two friends teamed up and without even realizing it set something powerful in motion. It's the story of how a simple plan to walk together each morning prompted life changes for both of us. Now more than six years later, when we turn around and realize how far we've gone together, we are amazed.

For example, in addition to training for and running the half marathon in 2003, today we:

- work out an average of five days a week, running, cycling, kickboxing, or weightlifting;
- have competed in several races this year alone, from local 10Ks to 5Ks;
- are training for our first marathon and will once again complete a half marathon, in preparation for the full distance;
- contemplate training for a duathlon or triathlon;
- can jump rope nonstop for fifteen minutes (and perhaps longer);
- have started eating healthier and paying closer attention to how our bodies use food and nutrients for fuel and performance;
- are more muscular and toned;
- have lost several inches and pounds, changed our figures dramatically, seen our weight stabilize, and wear smaller-sized clothes;
- have low blood pressure and healthy hearts;

- have seen positive medical results, such as a noticeable reduction in migraine occurrences and a quicker, easier recovery from surgery;
- are far more in tune with our bodies and our minds, and what we need in order for us to be at our best;
- are less emotional and more even-keeled;
- are less bothered by daily stressors, especially the little, everyday annoyances;
- don't worry and fret as much;
- sleep better and feel more rested;
- have more energy (and the ability) to keep up with our active boys;
- aren't afraid of physical or mental challenges;
- understand the ebbs and flows of motivation, focus, discipline, and how to get back on track when we become derailed;
- know how to set boundaries;
- understand ourselves better—what we like and what we don't, where we want to go in life and how to devise a plan to get there;
- walk with confidence;
- are good role models for our children by living an active, healthy lifestyle;
- consider ourselves athletes, in every sense of the word.

These types of accomplishments—and others—can become part of your life story too.

Inside these pages we hope to inspire you and a friend. We'll explain our philosophy and formula regarding how a regular exercise routine coupled with the power of friendship can stimulate a unique and forceful phenomenon.

We'll detail exactly what we did, how we did it, and how you can get started on your own journey. Each chapter will introduce you to a phase of ours. It will include our personal experiences from that time in our lives. We share our stories in each chapter because we believe it's likely there are parts of our journey that you might be able to identify with. Then you'll find a kind of "how-to" section, which contains practical advice, suggestions, tips, and guidance. At times, our advice mirrors the exact steps we took. Other times, our advice varies a bit from how we ventured forth, simply because in hindsight we realize there is a better way to proceed than the path we took. We will also help you understand what types of changes you can expect—from subtle to distinct changes in your body, your mind, and your spirit. Throughout, we hope to sprinkle inspiration and motivation to keep you going. Finally, and most important, we will continually focus on helping you nurture and use your partnership so that each of you is reaping the full benefits of your friendship and your time together.

Now, all you need to do is read on and discover how putting one foot in front of the other can alter your life forever.

THE BEST FRIENDS' GUIDE TO GETTING FIT

A BIRDSEYE VIEW

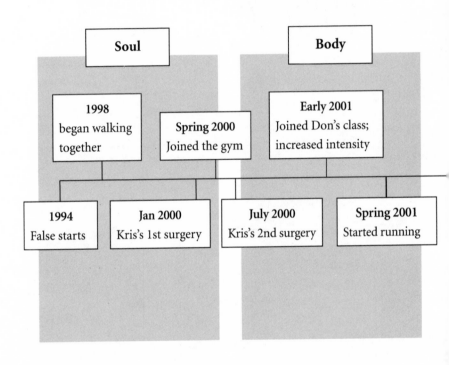

OF OUR JOURNEY

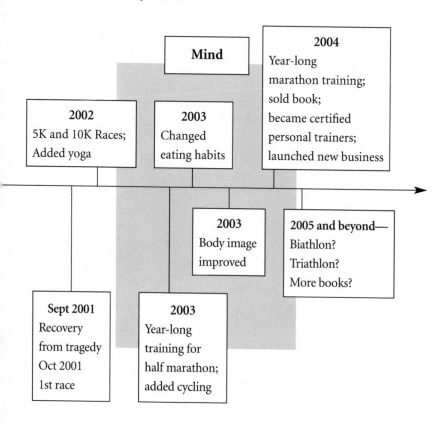

Mind

2004
Year-long
marathon training;
sold book;
became certified
personal trainers;
launched new business

2002
5K and 10K Races;
Added yoga

2003
Changed
eating habits

2003
Body image
improved

2005 and beyond—
Biathlon?
Triathlon?
More books?

Sept 2001
Recovery
from tragedy
Oct 2001
1st race

2003
Year-long
training for
half marathon;
added cycling

CHAPTER 1

OUR FORMULA FOR SUCCESS

I F YOU'VE READ our introductions, then you have a good idea of our personal struggles and a bit about where we are today. Do we have perfect, dream bodies? Nope (and we never will). Do we handle every situation with ease and patience? Hardly. Are we winning races, clinching titles, and breaking records? Not even close.

But on any given day, for the majority of our waking hours, we feel pretty good about ourselves. We feel athletic, strong, capable, balanced, in control, stable, confident, secure, accomplished, content, and optimistic.

Are there areas of our lives, our emotions, our bodies, we want to improve or change? Of course. There always will be. It's a lifelong pursuit and an ongoing process. Our approach to working out and staying fit is a fluid one. We have good days and bad. We have focused stretches of training time. We also have weeks when our workouts mostly support our need to socialize. There's an ebb and flow to staying fit.

It's important for you to realize (before you read any further) that this book is not a guide to achieving the ideal swimsuit body. It's not about becoming a marathon runner, an aerobics instructor, or triathlete. It's about finding your own balance and your strengths in whatever you choose to pursue, physically or otherwise. It's about learning to listen to your own inner voice for the knowledge of what you need, from pursuing your passions to engaging in an activity to choosing the foods that are right for you. It's about *becoming the best that you can be*, at any given moment, during the better part of your days. Finally, it's about finding a way to make yourself a priority within your own life and to give yourself the mental, physical, and emotional outlets and challenges that you require.

This chapter will outline our fundamental philosophy, which will form the foundation for your entire journey. It also includes a snapshot of our journey, from where we started to where we are today to where we think we're headed. We hope this snapshot will help you see how our focus on nurturing different elements of ourselves—body, mind, and soul—led to overall wellness, strength, and fitness.

Again, we can't say it enough: *if we can achieve it, you can achieve it.* No matter how many times in your life you may have tried and failed.

∼ A Bird's-Eye View of Our Journey ∼

Look at the chart on pages xxii and xxiii. This is a snapshot of our journey. If you look at it, from start to finish, in terms of fitness, it began as early as 1994 when we experienced some false starts and failures (which we'll explore further in a moment).

Our more successful kickoff occurred in 1998, simply enough, with a plan to walk together five days a week. That routine lasted for quite a while. In fact, you can see that it wasn't until a year and a half later that we tried anything other than walking. Throughout this book, we'll explore all of these phases in our journey including how we experienced some false starts, how and why we started walking together, how and why we moved on to joining a gym, how and why we started to increase the intensity of our workouts, how and why we began to blossom in terms of self-confidence, how and why we began to develop inner discipline to change our eating habits, and of course, how and why you can make similar changes in yourself and your life. You'll find that every chapter in the book mirrors a milestone on this time line.

You'll also notice that layered beneath the time line are the labels Soul, Body, and Mind. As we've said, we believe that to be fit means that your body, your mind, your soul fit together seamlessly, effortlessly, powerfully. They work together. They feel strong and empowered to help you become the best that you can be.

To achieve this, we believe you must begin by nurturing your soul as you move your body. Over time, as your soul becomes fulfilled and your body begins to enjoy movement, it will want to move more—more often and more intensely. As you feed this need and challenge yourself physically, you will also be challenging yourself mentally. That enables you to develop greater discipline, focus, and resolve. With that, you will find that your life decisions become more mindful, more purposeful, more controlled. When you reach that point, you will have the type of mental discipline and focus that is necessary to successfully make long-term changes in areas you may have previously struggled with—such as your eating habits or how you view your body. The labels show you which aspect (soul, body, mind) is being *exercised* during each phase of the journey.

∽ False Starts and Failures ∽

Before we outline our formula for success, let's look at the first entry on our time line: 1994 False Starts. It's important that we start here for two reasons. First, it illustrates that you can succeed no matter how many times you may have failed in the past. Second, it's important to compare what works with what doesn't.

In 1994, we were both pregnant. (We had become friends while dating our future husbands who were childhood friends.) Our due dates were within a couple weeks of each other and throughout the pregnancies, our friendship deepened. Here's how we remember that time and our failed attempts to get fit.

∾ Kris Looks Back ∾

I faced a host of health issues before becoming pregnant. As a result, I wanted to be sure that I maintained healthy habits throughout my pregnancy. Before I became pregnant, I had taken up running. But I didn't want to run during the pregnancy, so I was searching for another activity.

I found an aerobics class for pregnant women, taught by a prenatal nurse. Kim was interested in attending with me, so we both went together. We'd meet at the class, one night a week.

After Scotty was born life changed so dramatically. I remember that first Christmas, when he was only three months old. My husband gave me several gifts that consisted of workout attire and ski clothing. There were tight leggings and snow pants. While only a year earlier I would have relished getting all this gear, now I was a bit astounded to receive it. It seemed, already, so far removed from who I had become and who I was. I was a mom. That was my main focus.

There simply wasn't any time to exercise. Or so I thought. It probably didn't matter how many hours there were in a day, exercise just wasn't going to happen during any of them.

∾ Kim Looks Back ∾

Kris and I took a prenatal exercise class together, during my second pregnancy when my older son was just a little over a year old. I really can't remember why the idea of working out during pregnancy intrigued me. With a toddler at home, a home-based business, and my husband's business also operating out of the basement, I may have needed a simple outlet, something to get me out of the house for a time.

But it was definitely challenging to get out of the house to get to the classes. My husband was very supportive, but it required coordinating the logistics and making a concerted effort. After each class, I distinctly remember racing home as quickly as I could, not wanting to be gone any longer than necessary.

I enjoyed the class, but once my second son was born, the thought of exercise didn't cross my mind again for another several months, perhaps even years. I was in the throes of what I consider my most intense and draining time as a mommy, with two young children close in age. There were too many tasks to attend to and too little energy to do it all. Squeezing time in for myself was not a priority.

✎ Our Greatest Challenge ✎

It's easy to see that time—finding time, making time, taking time—was our earliest and greatest challenge. After the babies came, taking time for ourselves was not a consideration, let alone a priority. It was always the last item on our never-ending list of things to do. It seemed as if there were no time to take. We were starting to lose ourselves in the demands of our families (albeit willingly). With no routine established and no incentive for continuing on, fitness took a backseat to every other priority driving our lives.

✎ A Formula That Can Work for You ✎

When we kicked off our walking routine in 1998, two things were different from when we attended the prenatal exercise class together. First, we wrapped our friendship around the activity of walking. Second, we established a specific time for our routine. Those two differences have contributed to our ability to maintain a routine over several years and to succeed at changing our lives. These two points form the core of our entire philosophy and approach—it's our formula for success.

OUR FORMULA FOR SUCCESS is for you to

1. Get fit with a friend.
2. Get into a specific daily movement routine.

If you don't follow any other piece of advice in this entire book—if you take these pearls of wisdom to heart—we believe without a shadow of a doubt that you too can succeed.

Get Fit with a Friend

We believe in the power of friendship. We believe that the element of friendship and making a commitment to one another is what helps keep those false starts at bay. When we started walking in 1998, we were able to spend time connecting—nurturing our souls. We were reliant on one another to follow through. We became addicted to our time together. The exercise class, on the other hand, didn't provide that opportunity. We couldn't talk to each other during class, so we weren't connecting and nurturing our souls.

Think about your own false starts. Have they occurred largely because you were on your own, struggling for motivation, desire, structure, and incentive?

Having a friend to partner with helps curb waning desire and motivation. It gives you a reason to go. The friendship seduces you into being consistent, because more often than not, the reason you're going is to have a laugh and enjoy each other's company (rather than because you're looking forward to having a great walk). Being accountable to one another helps get you over a hump when you don't feel like being consistent. Hopefully, your motivation lags at different times. Still, even if a slump hits at the same time, it's much easier to weather it when you have a friend to commiserate with.

All of our own fitness achievements—together and independent of one another—are directly related to our partnership. Without argument, we could not have done this without each other. It is our partnership—our friendship—that has nurtured our emotional and spiritual sides, making them stronger. It is the friendship that has given us the incentive, time after time, to get up each morning and to get out the door to meet each other for a workout, no matter how much we'd rather not. The added mental toughness that comes from that follow-through has prompted us to (eventually and in due time) tackle greater physical challenges. It all goes hand in hand.

Get into a Specific, Daily Movement Routine

Picking a certain time each day to move your body will help ensure consistency in your routine. Life is too chaotic for exercise to be squeezed in whenever there's an open snippet of time. That time never comes. So you need to establish a set time and routine. For our walks, we chose the 5:30 a.m. time slot, Monday through Friday. With our hectic schedules, and between work, kids, husbands, and houses there was no other available time that we could claim for ourselves daily. Yet few things, other than an occasional business trip by our husbands, ever derailed that time together. Choosing your sacred time will be your single, greatest challenge.

What's important to note here, is that during our false start, the time period for the exercise class was chosen for us. Once the class was over, so was our routine. Whereas, with our early morning walking routine, the time remained the same. As our pursuits changed, and we took up activities like running, we still maintained our 5:30 a.m. routine. So pick your time first, then choose which activity works best. (In the next chapter, "Getting Started," we'll provide you with some additional points on how to pick a time that works for you and how to establish a routine.)

The combination of consistency and your ability to connect regularly with a friend is what will lead to success and to dramatic results in all areas of your life, from your emotional to your physical self—mind, body, and soul. Let's look at why this works.

❧ The Power of Friendship ❧

Think back to when you were a little girl. Remember how you and your best friend giggled together for hours? How you shared all your secrets? Remember how just knowing she was there for you made you feel stronger and more secure?

As women we may be older, but we still have a need to be giggling girlfriends. We are social beings. Friendships are a critical component of our overall mental well-being. Yet often, as we become professionals, wives, and mothers, we don't have time to connect on a regular basis with a close friend. Sure, we may make friends while standing guard at the playground. Or click with women at work. Or hang out together at the neighborhood block party. But it takes time and dedication to be a best friend. In today's frantic world, who can squeeze that in? So while we may share tips for potty training or for handling a prickly boss, we are not likely to engage in deeper, more personal discussions.

Yet we need those types of friendships and interactions—where we can discuss our dreams, aspirations, and fears—in order for us to be at our best emotionally.

As great as our marriages or committed relationships may be, there is a different dynamic between girlfriends that cannot be duplicated with spouses, fiancés, or boyfriends.

That's why the friendship component is so critical to our philosophy. Having an ongoing opportunity to nurture a best friendship will help you achieve a greater degree of mental, spiritual, and emotional fitness and stability.

It will transcend every aspect of your life—in ways you cannot quite comprehend today—including how you pursue becoming more physically fit. Besides, given the choice, wouldn't you just love to be able to spend between one and two hours a day with a best friend, chatting, laughing, and finding yourselves once again? Think of how good it would feel to do that, day after day, year after year, without feeling guilty.

∾ How to Pick a Partner ∾ You Can Succeed With

For this to work, however, you need to pick your partner wisely. This cannot be stressed enough. So take your time.

You may already have the perfect friend in mind. That's great. But if not, here are some points to consider:

Pick a Girlfriend

This is a must. You *must* choose a female friend. This is not the time to impress some beefcake at work. It's not an opportunity to have a platonic relationship that will lift you from the doldrums of your marriage. All of those male-female relationships will add too many complicated dimensions to your life (that we're not equipped to address). Trust us on this: stick with your own kind.

Consider Your Compatibility Quotient

What kind of person are you? Who or what kind of person do you mesh with best? To help determine this, think about your closest friends and the types of people they are. Are they similar to you? Or different from you? In what ways?

Try to find the type of woman that you naturally click with; that person you thoroughly enjoy and wish you could spend more time around. You may find that your first choice is someone you know pretty well, but you do not necessarily consider a best friend. That's okay. In time, your relationship will deepen.

Because you will spend large chunks of time with this person, also be sure it is someone you can be completely yourself with. Pick someone you trust. Choose a friend you can laugh with. Select a person you can rely on. Choose someone with whom you can have a healthy spirit of competition. (You want to be able to motivate each other and propel each other forward, but you should not be trying to outdo one another.) Most important, find an equal partner, someone with whom you can have a voice.

Become a Matched Set

It does not necessarily matter what stage of life you are in, but you should choose a friend who is at a similar stage. You may both be single professionals. Or, perhaps you both are married and have young children. Or, the two of you may be newly retired, empty nesters.

Regardless, being a matched set means you will have more chances to relate to each other in terms of your daily experiences, foibles, thoughts, and dreams. It will also be easier to find a common time to get together, if your schedules are dictated by similar types of commitments.

This general rule also applies to your fitness level. Find a partner who is in the same shape (or lack of shape) as you. If you haven't exercised in ten years, it makes no sense for you to partner with a competitive runner. You want to be in this together, not feeling like you're either being left behind or held back by your friend. By being at a similar fitness level, you will help inspire, motivate, and encourage one another. You will be able to laugh with each other when you feel winded and sore. You will also be able to revel in your accomplishments together.

Find Someone Close By

It will be easier to succeed if your partner lives nearby. Walking distance is ideal, but driving distance is workable. You will have to work out the logistics. You may choose to meet some place in between your two homes (such as a bike path, a walking trail, a school, a gym, or a track). Or, you may decide that each week one friend will drive to the other's home so you can stroll the neighborhood.

Once you've picked your partner, you will have to approach her with your ideas. (Consider buying her a copy of this book to help her see the light!) Good luck. But don't get discouraged if she declines. Just put your thinking cap on and find another friend. As soon as the two of you are committed, then you're ready to get started.

∾ Notes ∾

Jot down the names of women you know (who may or may not be close friends of yours today) who might be good candidates for becoming your partner.

Think about each one on the list. What do you like about the person? What concerns do you have about partnering with her? Write down some pros and cons for each. One might live right next door (pro) while another lives across town (con).

CHAPTER 2

GETTING STARTED

EVERY NEW ADVENTURE begins somewhere. This chapter will present the basics on how you can begin your journey, including what you and your partner need to consider as you set up your own personal routine, what you can expect to encounter in terms of challenges and benefits, and how you can overcome your own past failures and false starts.

We were talking the other day, trying to remember exactly how this journey of ours began. In light of all our past failures and attempts to diet and exercise, it's hard to believe that it began at all, let alone that we've actually finally succeeded. It was so unplanned, so unstructured, that it took us a while to remember how it came to be.

∼ Kim Looks Back ∼

In late 1997, I caught an episode of the *Oprah Winfrey Show* featuring Sarah Ban Breathnach discussing her book *Simple Abundance*. With its subtitle, *A Daybook of Comfort and Joy*, it sounded intriguing. I had joy, but needed a bit of comfort.

I had been stretching myself as thin as humanly possible in an effort to attain what I had been raised to believe: that a woman can have it all.

When I was growing up, my mom (who was divorced) had a powerful and demanding career at a time when most women—especially mothers—did not work. I spent a fair amount of my childhood either in day care settings, with babysitters, or alone at home after school. While it certainly was a misperception on my part, I believed for a long time that her career was her number one priority.

My husband, on the other hand, had been raised in a far more traditional manner by a stay-at-home mom. So, while we came to the task of child rearing from completely different perspectives, we agreed on one thing: that I would stay home with the kids, although it did not necessarily mean that I would also step away from my career. After all, I had been raised (not just by my mother, but by our entire society) to believe I could have it all, that I could do it all. The notion of stepping away from my career would have meant a clear and utter failure on my part to be all that a woman should be. So, while it was critically important for me to be home with the kids, I was bound and determined to find a way to continue to work.

Thus, I worked overtime trying to balance being a stay-at-home mom with running a freelance writing business. My husband, who also ran a business out of the home, was incredibly supportive. Often, we used a tag-team approach. He would be with the boys while I scrambled to get some work done, and vice versa.

But I was horrible at turning down assignments, and as a result, often took on more work than I could realistically handle. That required me to become a master at developing creative solutions for getting everything done. I awoke each morning at 5 a.m. to work until the kids woke up at 7 a.m. I worked while they napped. If my husband wasn't available to help, I would participate in conference calls while huddled in the bathroom, phone in hand, with the fan whirring in the background in an effort to drown out their playful squeals and shrieks. I often worked late into the night and on weekends in order to meet deadlines. I ran down to check my e-mail when *Barney* was on and proofread documents while they ate their Mac and cheese lunches.

For me, it seemed well worth all the juggling. Yet the grueling schedule took its toll. As the boys were moving through their toddler and preschool years, my husband sold his business and changed careers. That meant he was gone from the house each day, and so I wasn't able to rely on him to help me juggle the workload. Yet, I didn't take on any less work.

And so, by the time the boys were three and five, I was feeling overwhelmed and in need of some soothing comfort.

That's when I stumbled upon the Oprah show and Ban Breathnach's appearance. Since Kris and I had often talked about the struggle to balance our family lives and our work commitments, I felt she might enjoy the book too. I bought us each a copy of *Simple Abundance* that Christmas (1997). Filled with daily essays of inspiration, the book offers thought-provoking ideas surrounding the concept of living a meaningful, purposeful, rich, yet simple life.

On January 1, 1998, we began to read one essay each day. We found her words pushed us to be more introspective and to think about ourselves—our likes, dislikes, sense of style, purpose, and hobbies. Not only did her words speak to us, they resonated loudly, because we had spent so little time thinking about such ideas.

∼ Kris Looks Back ∼

During the spring of 1998, when my son was three years old, we started to plan a move to a larger home. We found one located right around the corner from Kim.

That was the year I had received *Simple Abundance* as a gift from her. We were both reading the daily essays and talking about it frequently. Ban Breathnach was a huge advocate the notion that you should fill your life with all the things you love. She extended that philosophy to everything—from the type of furniture you picked, to the types of hobbies you pursued, to how you earned your living. Her approach seemed almost decadent compared to our own more self-sacrificing approach.

How had we gotten to that place? Where thinking about ourselves seemed as if it were self-indulgent?

To analyze how you arrive at a place in life, you often have to look back at your role models and your upbringing. For me, that means looking to my mother. At the tender age of nineteen, she got married, then bore three children and divorced all in a period of nine years. Following the divorce she put herself through school, had a nursing career, and raised the three of us. She never had anyone clean her house, wash her car, or take care of her lawn—except, of course, her children.

As a result, when I became pregnant I never considered giving up my career. I distinctly remember having an explicit conversation with my mom, in which I stated that I was willing to give up everything else—exercising, reading books, and socializing with friends—in order to have my career, my husband, and our new baby. She validated my choice.

In fact, that's essentially what I did. The first year of my son's life I worked part-time in the office and part-time at home. By the end of his first year, I somehow managed to be promoted. Over the next two years, I held a big job at work, and an equally big job at home. I dressed in power suits by day and mommy smocks by night, but neither outfit suited me very well.

I really had no identity of my own. Things were so blandly me, that even all the walls in my house were painted white. They were white because I didn't even know what color I liked. Moreover, I had no time to care. Yet I convinced myself that I preferred white walls, rather than admitting that I had picked that "color" by default.

So, when we began to read *Simple Abundance*, it caused me to ask such questions as "What are my favorite colors? Why are all my walls white?"

At the end of each month's section of essays, Ban Breathnach included a checklist of items to buy, adventures to try, and things to consider. For example, the list of "Joyful Simplicities for January" included:

- Go through your personal papers at home and organize your desk to get a fresh start on the New Year.
- Visit an art supply shop and simply look around. Take in all the different ways you can begin to express yourself.
- Visit the local library and read some new magazines you don't normally subscribe to.
- Prepare for a winter's idyll. Stock the pantry with real cocoa, tiny marshmallows, and a bar of good chocolate.

We loved the fact that the book gave us permission to care for—and almost pamper—ourselves. It was an act that we had intentionally chosen not to do because of our focus on our families and careers. Many of her ideas we embraced, while others had us scratching our heads and wondering, "Who has time for that?"

On April 16, 1998, just a couple of months before our move, we read her essay "Walking as Meditation." Here is an excerpt:

As long as I approached walking as exercise I never made it past the front door. But one day I felt so anxious I felt as if I would jump out of my skin, and so I bolted out of the house at lunchtime as if I were leaving the scene of a crime. Filled with disappointments, painful memories, and my own unrealistic expectations from the past—terrified of what the future held and the changes that were inevitable—the only safe place for me was the present moment: my foot against the pavement, the wind on my face, my breath entering and leaving my body. Forty minutes later I stopped, discovered to my amazement that I was on the other side of town, and headed back home, calm and centered. I have been walking ever since.

Slowly I am learning what Henry David Thoreau knew: "It requires a direct dispensation from Heaven to become a walker." But I still don't walk for exercise. Instead, I walk regularly for my soul and my body tags along.

Shortly after that day, we were loading boxes and moving into our new home. Those words of comfort, the idea of walking and using it as a form of meditation, struck a chord with both of us. While we didn't feel the need to bolt out of our houses, we did yearn to be calm and centered. Somehow we decided that we could combine several of Sarah's pieces of advice and that we would walk together. But we knew that we had to do it early in the morning before our families awoke.

And that's how our routine began.

∿ Putting One Foot in Front of the Other ∿

Our initial plan was to meet on the corner in between our two houses and walk together. We had no goals, no dreams, no strategy, and no clue. Our only intention was to meet five days a week (Monday through Friday) in the wee morning hours. It's almost amazing that we followed through. But we did. We still remember that first day. Right at the beginning of our walk was a small hill. At a snail's pace we started forth. By the time we reached the top (which was about a block and a half away) we were winded. Thankfully, we were both huffing and puffing equally. It made us chuckle that we were so out of shape.

That first day we walked roughly one mile.

It was a start. And a good one at that. The next day our muscles were sore. That showed us that we had accomplished something, no matter how small.

After a few weeks, we found we were less and less winded going up the hill. Still, we kept our pace comfortable, slow, and casual. We were having the best time talking and laughing and enjoying the quiet freshness of the early mornings. We walked the same route for months, almost a full year.

∾ How to Start Your Walking Plan ∾

OK. You and your friend have decided to commit to each other and to a plan. Now what? The rest of this chapter outlines how to get started. If you and your friend believe you're ready for something other than a walking program, read this chapter anyway. You may find some tips that still apply. Then thumb through subsequent chapters and explore where a good starting point for you might be. Remember, your initial focus is on connecting as friends while you're moving your body. So, whichever activity you choose, it should support your ability to chat with one another. That might be slow-to-moderate jogging or using side-by-side elliptical trainers or stationary bikes. Whatever you choose, use it as your license to gab. (As with starting any exercise program, you should first consult your physician.)

∾ Taking that First Step ∾

If you haven't exercised in years, don't worry about how fast or how far you're going. Instead, simply set a goal to get together to walk three to five days a week.

Then plan to cherish your time together. Your primary focus should be nurturing your friendship as well as feeding your souls with laughter and meaningful moments.

Most important, take the pressure off of yourselves "to perform" or to reach a set of goals. Forget your vision of where you want to be someday—whether that means at some ideal weight or fulfilling a personal fantasy of yourself. Again, your only goal at this point should be to try to walk with your friend three to five times each week and in doing so, establish a routine. Recognize that by walking, and doing it regularly, you are probably doing more than you did last month, or last year, or the last five years. You're headed in the right direction.

∼ Establishing a Routine ∼

In order to establish your routine, you'll need to decide:

- where to meet regularly
- when to meet regularly

Depending upon where you and your friend live in relation to one another, you may decide to meet halfway between your homes (either by walking to get there or by driving). Or, perhaps there is a school nearby that has a track where you can walk. Or, a beautiful park that's not too far. While it's great to be creative in terms of finding a lovely place to walk, initially the more critical factor is whether or not the spot is convenient for both of you. If it's not convenient, you won't be able to be consistent.

Deciding *when* to meet and coordinating your schedules may be an even trickier task. It may require lots of dialogue and comparing calendars. Plan to get together and compare your day planners, so that you can see when there are chunks of time that you both have available. If you absolutely can't find any chunks of time, then you need to *make* time for yourselves.

Because our schedules were so hectic, we decided to meet at the corner at 5:30 in the morning. Logistically it made sense. It was the only time we would be able to commit to regularly. (Looking back, it was a brilliant idea because no matter how intense the daily grind of activities got, few things ever interrupted our time together. That's still true today.)

If you have children, you may also find it easier to get out, do your walk, and return home before anyone wakes up. In the early morning, you probably won't have to grapple with soliciting support from your husband or a babysitter, and you won't infringe on other family members' schedules. The early morning hours can also work well because it's difficult to call someone to cancel unless it's a dire emergency, for fear you'll wake up the entire household. That can be a great incentive for getting up and out the door.

While scheduling the time at the crack of dawn may be easiest, waking up and getting out of bed never is. Even today, it's never easy for us to get out of bed—even all these years after having established our routine. Just do it.

If your husband travels frequently or you work a shift, the mornings may not be realistic. Talk to your friend openly about what time(s) work best for both of you. While getting together the same time each day may be ideal, be prepared to be flexible. Arrive at a solution that works for both. If that means four late nights and middays on Thursdays, go for it!

Once you've picked your time slot, guard it with your life. Depending upon which time you choose, you may find there are 101 priorities suddenly clamoring for that exact same moment. Protect your time vigilantly. Learn to say, "No I'm sorry, I can't do that . . . I have an appointment." (If you had an appointment with a doctor, you would juggle the other commitments long before you would call to reschedule with the doctor. Treat this appointment with the same respect and reverence.) Think of it this way: *you will not succeed if you cannot get together regularly*. Find a way to succeed.

Unfortunately, the person who may encroach upon your time most may be your husband. This is a delicate issue. He may start to see that you're on to something. He may envy your time. He may even try to schedule his own pursuit for that same time slot. Don't be surprised to hear, "I'm going to play tennis with Ralph tomorrow at 7:00." Resist the urge to pounce. While you may have to relinquish your time on that particular day, be sure you impress upon him the importance of this time for you. In this or any instance, it's hard for us as women to put ourselves first and to be "selfish" with our wants and needs. Stand firm. It will prove beneficial to everyone if you do. In the long run, your kids will benefit. Your husband will benefit. Your boss and peers will benefit. Of course, you will benefit too. It's a win-win solution if you can make it work. If you find that conflicts keep arising and you are not getting the support you need, pick a different time—be it at the crack of dawn or the stroke of midnight. There are twenty-four hours in each day. You deserve at least one of those for yourself!

∾ **Making Yourself a Priority** ∾

Making time for yourself means you need to make yourself a priority in your own life. This could be your next greatest challenge. It's so easy for us as women to put our needs on the back burner. It's easy to trick ourselves into thinking that everyone else's needs come before our own. It's easy to forget we even have needs. However, while you must make sacrifices for the good of your family, your career, or a needy parent, you do not have to sacrifice yourself. There is a difference.

That is another reason why waking up before the crack of dawn works well for us. Mentally, we do not feel that we are taking anything away from our families or their needs. No one even really notices that we're not at home. We've managed to carve time out for ourselves without having an impact on the children or our husbands. We can do it without feeling guilty. We can do it without worrying about logistics. Again, as difficult as it may be to rouse yourself at such an ungodly hour, it is certainly an ideal way to address adding yourself to the list of priorities without taking away from anyone or anything else. Making yourself a priority means you are willing to wake up early even though you're bone tired, because you know you're worth the struggle of getting out of bed.

If you are a new mother, or a single mom, or if you have very young children at home, it may seem as if the last thing you can or want to do is get up any earlier than you already do. That's fair, for now. But consider finding another mom in the neighborhood whom you can meet with your kids and your strollers. It may not be the ideal solution, but it is certainly a step in the right direction. It will get you both moving, talking, and connecting. As your children get older you will be able to refine your approach and your schedule. The key initially will be making yourself enough of a priority so that you can achieve frequency within your routine.

If one or both of you has a demanding job and you find you are both traveling a lot, consider chatting on a cell phone while you both walk in separate cities. Or, take a journal with you and jot down thoughts that come to mind on your independent walks, then compare notes when you are both home again.

Be creative and committed. After all, if you don't care for you, then who else will? Someday you'll look back and wonder how it is exactly that you fell off the list of top priorities in your own life!

⟶ **The Beauty of a Routine** ⟵

The beauty of a routine is that you know exactly what to expect. Strive to create a routine that is mindlessly automatic. Meet at the same place at the same time (based on your schedules.) Lay out your clothes the previous night (or day), including everything you'll need—from shoes to socks to a jacket. Don't push the snooze button repeatedly. Wear the same basic clothes. If you're getting up early, get a coffee maker that will brew coffee on a timer basis, so it's ready when you wake up. Leave your house at the same time. Follow the same route on your walks.

Getting into a routine is also made easier by having a partner because you will be accountable to someone. She is relying on you. Knowing she's waiting for you at some designated point—perhaps beneath a cold, dark sky—will be a huge motivator on those (many) days when you don't feel like going. It's difficult to blow off a friend and not expect repercussions.

So don't call to cancel unless you're sick and can't get out of bed. Every once in a while, we found that one of the kids would be so sick that, having been up all night, we would be unable to get up the next morning for our walk. If you have to break your routine because of an illness or a vacation, *get back on track immediately*. Just assume you will start back up again as soon as the interruption is over. Then follow through.

Perhaps most critical to establishing your routine is this: don't reward yourself by taking a day off. This rewards the wrong behavior. If you need to pat yourselves on the back for being consistent, treat yourselves to something special after your walk (like a Starbucks coffee).

Finally and perhaps obviously, once your routine is established, don't vary it.

⟶ **Through Wind, Rain, and Snow—** ⟵ **Staying Consistent**

If you're walking outside, you will occasionally encounter bad weather. Prepare for it. Check the weather report each night, so you know what to expect. Don't skip your walks because it's nasty outside—unless there is a torrential downpour or driving snow. Since consistency is critical, you must find a way to walk despite the weather.

The only time we skipped our walks because of weather was if we feared there would be ice on the roads (given the darkness at that hour, it's hard to spot ice and we didn't want to take a tumble). But those were generally the only times we missed, aside from major storms. If you live in a part of the country that sees more snow or rain than we do in Virginia, you may have to be more creative in order to be consistent. Consider meeting during the winter months at an area mall, parking garage, or health club. Or, buy those slip-on ice spikes that you can pull over the souls of your sneakers.

To combat the cold, be sure to bundle up and wear layers. Invest in the proper gear and clothing so you'll be comfortable. We wore layers of long johns, sweats, socks, and windpants. We sported raincoats, winter coats, gloves, and hats. We even enjoyed our discussions of what gear we would need based on the season. "Have you tried ear muffs?" we might ask.

If you can be consistent—*and you can*—you will experience your first boon in confidence. Why? Because you will be able to look back and point to a very specific accomplishment: *sticking to your routine despite the wind, rain, snow, or cold.* It will prove to you and to others that you are committed and that you can follow through. That's a huge achievement. Be proud of yourselves for that. And realize that if you can do this, you can master other challenges, too.

Friends, coworkers, and peers who learn of your accomplishment will greet you with surprise and envy. Whenever people learned that we walked regularly at 5:30 in the morning through the bad weather winter months, they were impressed. That made us feel good!

Each day that you add to your total tally of days spent walking means it will be harder for you to quit your program and easier for you to continue. It's a building process and you are completing your foundation for improved fitness.

So, hang in there. And think of us. No matter where you live or what time of year it may be, we are still getting up each and every morning, stumbling downstairs to our coffee cups, grabbing our water bottles, and heading out to meet each other. And we're hoping that you're doing the same.

∼ **What We Found, What You Can Expect** ∼

Initially, the benefits we experienced from walking together were primarily felt in our hearts and in our souls. Here's what we discovered:

- Having a regular outlet to discuss what's on your mind helps re-
  lieve stress. When you always have someone to turn to, virtually
  every day, stress doesn't have a chance to build and peak to unhealthy levels.
- No matter your age or stage in life, there will be life moments,
  events, or decisions that will consume your attention. Maybe you
  will face a move, new job, failing marriage, infertility, infidelity,
  the death of a loved one, an illness, or a crisis. Having this time
  and a sounding board will enable you to sort things out, privately
  and with a friend. That can bring you solace as well as help you
  shape your thoughts and decisions.
- Each time you get together, you'll feel as if you've accomplished
  something. Because you have. This feeling is enhanced when you
  walk first thing in the morning, since you'll feel as if you've completed something before most other people are even awake.

> For years, I had problems sleeping. I would toss and turn all night
> long. When we started walking, I noticed that on those days, I
> would sleep soundly the entire night. Even now on Sundays—
> when I don't generally work out—I will sleep restlessly, tossing
> and turning all night.
>
> —Kim

- With regular walking (or any exercise) you'll notice that you
  sleep better and more soundly at night. Getting a good night's
  rest (which can be a huge struggle for many people) is critical
  to a sense of well-being throughout the day. It affects your
  ability to cope, to be patient, to think clearly, and to enjoy life's
  moments.

- The partner approach provides a nice blend of private time and together time. We found that in the time it took to meet each other and then in our time walking back home, we were able to collect our thoughts regarding the day ahead. This seemed almost meditative in nature. Being able to get organized mentally will help you feel more in control of your days.
- Laughter is the best medicine. When you have the chance to either start your day with a laugh or decompress with a friend after a long day, you will feel more relaxed, lighter, and uplifted.
- If your children are very little, you may crave spending more time with adults. Your walks will provide you with that adult interaction as well as the chance to deepen a friendship.
- You can help bring out the best in each other. We have found that we have the ability to motivate each other time and time again to get things done, to tackle obstacles, to try new things, to be the best that we can be. Whether that means inspiring each other to be more disciplined in our eating habits or prompting each other to register for a race. Part of it is that we're competitive by nature. We don't want to be left behind—or worse—to have one succeed while the other fails. The end result is that we keep each other on track in terms of priorities. We keep each other moving forward in life.
- Because every day can be hectic, we found that when we walked in the mornings and returned before the kids awoke, we were able to start our days without feeling rushed—or worse—feeling as if we were already behind before the day had even begun.

These are just some of benefits we enjoyed. The list continues to grow as we take on new and different challenges (and we'll outline them in the following chapters).

Apart from the long list of benefits, there was one downside to our routine. While waking up early was the best solution for our schedules, the flip side to that solution was feeling tired. We found that in the late afternoons we'd hit a wall and be totally exhausted for an hour or so. On a rare occasion, we even dozed off in inappropriate places like the carpool line. By Thursday nights, we'd be so tired that we'd crawl into bed around 8:30 right after we tucked our kids in for the night. This lasted for a long, long time. Thankfully, we adjusted (although not for a couple of years).

If mornings are your sacred time, you need to accept the fact that there will be times when you will be tired—moments in every single day. But when you review the long list of benefits you will reap, it's a relatively small price to pay.

For your husband, however, having a sleepy wife may not fit the master plan. Your spouse needs to understand that, despite this, you still need the time. He needs to understand that eventually your body will adjust. Again, stand firm on keeping your commitment and work through it the best you can. Hopefully he will be patient. (If you're lucky, like we were, your spouses may also be friends. It certainly helped for each of our husbands to know that they weren't the only ones putting up with a snoring sweetheart.)

∾ It Becomes an Addiction ∾

Long before you ever become hooked on walking, you'll start to feel addicted to the time you and your friend spend together. It happens subtly and in stages. Initially, you get hooked on your chat time. You may also become addicted to having time that solely belongs to the two of you. It's a time when you can be totally and completely yourselves. You'll also notice and enjoy a deep and growing intimacy between you. Most important, you'll get addicted to the achievement and sense of accomplishment in getting together regularly.

Eventually, you'll notice that if you don't get your walk in, you miss it and are anxious for the next day. When "blowing it off" no longer feels like something you want to do, you'll know you're hooked.

∾ The Reactions of Others ∾

Even now years after our established routine, it feels good to see and hear how people react once they learn what we do. That was perhaps one of the earliest signs to us that we were on to something. That's because most people do not commit to regular exercise, though they may long to. An even larger portion of the population would never consider waking up before dawn to do it. So, when people learn that you follow through on such a commitment, especially in light of how hectic life can be, they marvel. That alone is a huge incentive—knowing that *you're already doing something that 90 percent of people would never do. Who cares if you're "just walking", they're still not even doing that!* And even if people like the idea and want to follow your lead, they won't. Few will ever put forth the effort that you are.

> I would be sitting at work, yawning, during a meeting and people would ask, "Up late last night?"
>
> I'd say, "No, I walk early in the morning."
>
> They'd ask, "How early?"
>
> When I'd respond "Five thirty a.m.," they'd say, "Wow!"
>
> I loved those reactions (and still do)!
>
> —Kris

You will also find that in addition to envying your commitment and dedication, people will envy the time that you share together. Some will feel the need to knock what you do, to discount your achievements, or to make excuses for why they don't do the same. Don't let them get to you. Just chat about it with your friend on your next walk. All of this will fuel your courage to protect your time even more and to continue on your journey.

Throughout the coming days, weeks, and years, remind yourself that you are accomplishing something that few others will. Praise yourself for that.

∽ A More Structured Walking Program ∽

We believe that you can start your journey without any goal other than to meet each other regularly (three to five times a week) for a walk. However, you may crave a bit more structure to get started. If so, here's a program that outlines how you can approach a walking program in a more methodical way.

Week 1: Start with a ten- to fifteen-minute walk at an easy pace. You should be able to carry on a comfortable conversation, without feeling winded. Walk three to five days the first week. Again, building your routine is your primary goal, so consistency is important.

Week 2: Add three to five minutes of walking a day, up to twenty minutes.

Week 3: Add three to five minutes a day, up to twenty-five minutes.

Week 4: Add three to five minutes a day, up to thirty minutes.

Once you are up to thirty minutes a day, walking three to five times a week, you can begin to pick up your pace a bit each day. This will allow you to cover more distance within the same amount of time and increase the challenge.

∼ Tips ∼

1. If you find walking for the suggested amount of time to be too difficult, cut back on the number of minutes, then repeat that schedule for another week or two, until you are able to progress comfortably.

2. Increase the time you spend walking each week before you increase your walking speed.

3. Be a good partner. If your partner feels aches and pains, slow down the pace and don't be in a rush to "achieve" a certain milestone.

4. As you walk, be aware of your posture. Think of lengthening your body with your head up, ears positioned over your shoulders, and your eyes forward. Hold your shoulders down and back, yet relaxed. Imagine tucking your shoulder blades into your back pocket. Tighten your abs and your gluts, and engage your muscles as you stride.

5. Your "rest" days are as important as your activity days.

6. Be sure to drink plenty of water before, during, and after your walk.

7. You should begin every walk with a slow warm-up. This means a slow-paced walk for three minutes or so. You can also add

some gentle stretching after your warm-up and before the main portion of your walk. (For stretching ideas, see appendix B, "Posture and Activity: Tips and Techniques.")

8. Remember on your walks to enjoy the moments. Check out the homes' landscaping. Notice the critters on your block. Enjoy the scent of the dew on the grass. Listen to crackles of the leaves and crunching of twigs beneath your feet. Best of all, listen to the giggles and squeals of laughter coming from you and your friend.

∾ How Long? ∾

It's hard to put a specific time frame on how many months you should continue your walking routine. You and your friend need to reach this decision together. It's not something you can decide today. Your positive results may prompt you to try something new, like running. Or, you may choose to never change your routine. Maybe you'll walk for one year. Maybe you'll walk forever.

Remember this: *walking every day is a great accomplishment!*

It took us more than a year before we considered doing anything different. We were not focused on the physical exercise aspect of our partnership. Instead, we were enjoying the time to ourselves and the idea that not many other people were doing what we were doing.

At some point you may choose to branch out and try something other than walking. You'll both know when it is time to pick up the pace or to try a new activity. One of you may take the lead and initiate the idea; just make sure the other one is ready to come along on the journey. If it's the right thing for you and your friend to do, it should feel as if it's a natural progression.

At a minimum though, we would suggest walking for one full year. That takes you through an entire cycle of weather, illnesses, and interruptions. Getting to the one-year mark will prove to you (and everyone else!) that you *can* be consistent. By then, your friendship will have deepened and it's likely you will be unwilling to give up what you have. You will be fully entrenched in your routine and will have the confidence to continue or to try something new.

Notes

With your partner, figure out the days and the times that work best for each of you. Where is there overlap? Where can you carve out a routine? Then brainstorm some ideas for *where* you can meet. Address how you will handle issues such as bad weather, sick kids, or a last minute glitch in the routine. Take notes on your decisions. After you begin, jot down what's working well and ideas for refining your routine.

CHAPTER 3

THE ART OF BEING
A BEST FRIEND

As women, we instantly understand the concept of a best friend. As a kid you may have had one special best friend or you may have cultivated many best friendships along the way. Interestingly, even though friendships often play an important role in childhood, as we age we have less and less time to devote to the proper care and feeding of a best friendship. Yet they are no less important to our overall mental well-being and health. Clearly, we are passionate about the critical role friendship has played in our journey. That's why we are zealous in our belief that each and every woman should have regular—even daily—doses of a deep and personal friendship. That may sound to you like an indulgence, but quite the contrary, we think it's as important as any other self-care ritual you may follow—from brushing your teeth to eating healthy foods. When you are able to wrap your friendship around an exercise routine, the rewards are innumerable.

Given we're grown women now, there are different tenets to this kind of friendship as opposed to the rules and structure we used as kids. Gone are the days of chanting, "I'll be your best friend," in order to manipulate someone into doing what you wanted them to do. (Though sometimes it might be nice if we could still wield that kind of power!) Gone are the days when you'd dress alike, in the same color, to show your allegiance to one another. And gone are the nightly, marathon phone calls to catch up on what happened after you left each other's company just an hour before.

Yes, grown-up friendships are a bit more sophisticated. So, how can you be tried and true friends, of the adult variety? This chapter explores the art of being best friends.

∿ Kris Looks Back ∿

This is so hard. I know Kim will have wonderful words and clever sentences to describe our friendship, and I so much want to be able to do the same thing. I want people to know and understand how important our friendship is to me and the balance it provides in my life. Have you ever read the book *The Red Tent*? In it, the women would gather each month during their menstrual cycle in a tent. For those few days, the women would pamper, listen to, and help each other. Their days were spent bonding with and enjoying each other's company, with no other distractions or concerns. I remember thinking, "OK, this is what modern women are missing today: time to bond with other women without distraction or interruption."

Kim and I created a similar environment, minus the red tent, during our morning walks. The time we spent together without distraction allowed us to learn and love so much about each other.

As young children we all had more time for friendships. But because of our jobs, husbands, and children, many of us have lost the time needed to devote to friendships as we have become women. I know I had lost having this type of connection with another woman for quite a while.

Looking back, I had past friendships that I would label as the best-friends kind. My first best friend was in grade school. We did everything together. I have such fond memories of the times we spent—practicing gymnastics in her basement night after night, wearing the same outfits in different colors. I often wonder about her. When I went off to college and moved away from my hometown, she stayed at home. As our interests became different, we lost touch.

Another woman whom I would consider a best friend was my college buddy. Time and proximity have prevented us from being able to connect on a regular basis. Then there was another close friend I had for a long time—through college, marriage, and my first baby—who was from my hometown but the relationship ended abruptly. I had angered her and she was not able to forgive me.

I cherish every one of my past friendships, but they were from my childhood.

As for my adult friendship with Kim, I can only say: it's perfect

"Are you two sisters?" people ask.

"Ha! Ha! Ha!" We laugh, "Do we really look alike?"

I have a European look, with big legs and shoulders, light skin, eyes, and hair. Kim looks Latina with slender arms and legs, dark skin, eyes, and hair. We do not look alike. So what is it that people see? What is it that we miss? Have we grown so close that we now resemble one another?

So, how exactly did we get so close? We've spent hours listening to one another. And we love each others' stories! We often laugh that when we're in a crowd no one else ever hears us speak—we are so soft spoken, our voices seem to always get drowned out. Except that we are always ready to listen to each other, often serving as the only person in the crowd to hear the telling of our friend's tale.

It's an easy friendship. She has always respected my need for privacy, never prying beyond what I want to share. And never would any of our conversations be shared with any other person. It requires no work for us to be friends.

So, how does one find such a friend? Willingness to dedicate some time to get to know someone beyond the obvious stuff. Kim and I have much in common to start with—husbands who grew up together, divorced parents, boys the same age. These commonalities helped us begin the friendship. The walks allowed us to really get to know each other. Now I feel so blessed and fortunate to have a great husband, a beautiful son, and a perfect friend. I can ask for no more.

∼ Kim Looks Back ∼

Growing up an only child in a divorced household can get a bit lonely. As far back as I can remember I turned to friends to fill the space where siblings and a larger family might normally be. I can remember many, many best friends throughout the years. At various points in my life, my friends were the single most important thing in the world to me.

As I got older, that only magnified. In my late teens, throughout college, and then in my early twenties, my closest girlfriends became my extended family. I'd spend endless hours with different friends, sharing intimate details of our lives as well as numerous adventures and hair-raising experiences. Five or so of those friendships still carry on today, though certainly time, distance, and commitments mean we only get to see and talk with each other occasionally (and sometimes rarely). Yet we're connected by a special bond of memories and a deep love for one another.

A few years after college, however, I felt some deep betrayals by friends I had held near and dear. Also within the same general time period, I had a couple of very close friends move far away. Perhaps because I put so much stock in friendships, those pains hit deeper than they might otherwise or should have. All of that, combined with the fact that I always felt abandoned by my dad, prompted me to learn how to better shield my heart. I became more guarded—but not on the surface. I still cultivated a host of new friends and developed a slew of relationships—many of whom I sincerely cared for, but I became a master at creating a sense of intimacy while still protecting myself from vulnerability and harm.

Because I was a good listener, I had a bad habit of playing therapist for my friends. With that technique, and without them even realizing it, I was easily able to keep them at bay, just beyond the point where they'd gain a true foothold on my heart. That allowed me to enjoy the relationships on my terms, and oddly enough, to feel relatively unphased if the relationship changed, dissipated, or ended altogether. Unfortunately, that sometimes created a lopsided imbalance in the relationships (where I'd know much about the person and she felt incredibly close to me, though she really knew little, if anything, about me). While it's hard to admit, it even became easy for me to slyly, subtly disconnect from relationships, if it made sense for me to do so. Always, I still relied on my handful of tried-and-true lifelong friends and, of course, on my husband to feed my need for closeness.

Although a few women nearly succeeded, Kris is the only one over the past decade or more to have fully cracked that hard, protective shell guarding my heart. So, how did she break through? Certainly much has to do with the sheer amount of time we spend together, but I never would have been able to spend that much time with just anyone. In the beginning, we became fast friends because we had so much in common. Our approach to life and to situations was so similar. We could relate to each other because of what we'd been through as kids. Since we are both intensely private people, we seemed to know how to let each other in while still respecting each other's need to hold back.

What lies at the core of our ability to connect more deeply is that give and take. There's a willingness we both have to listen, to ask questions, and to remember what matters to the other person. We genuinely care. We help each other explore, brainstorm, complain, and question, without passing judgment. We share the airtime, trading stories, listening intently, back and forth with ease. We confide in each other, understanding that at times, we may be the only other person on earth who will ever hear that utterance. We protect each other's privacy, never betraying trusts. We never, ever gossip about each other. We are fiercely loyal. All of that delivers a tremendous sense of faith and trust in one another and in our friendship. We believe in each other and in our partnership. And we're still growing closer, year after year. We've even reached new depths just while writing this book.

Perhaps the most unique aspect of our friendship versus any other one that I've had is that it's marked by such positive, meaningful pursuits. With other friendships, the interactions usually center around social gatherings or job situations. Yet our partnered fitness journey means that together we are growing and changing, setting goals, making plans, and empowering ourselves to reach heights we never thought possible. It means we share some incredible life-changing moments that add an underlying depth, bond, and purpose to our friendship. In all of these ways, it's unlike any other friendship I've ever had.

∼ Watching Your Friendship Grow ∼

Like any relationship, there's a certain chemistry or spark that has to happen between two people in order for them to become good friends. You have to click. Beyond that, building a good friendship can happen in hundreds of different ways.

So make no mistake, you don't need to start out on your journey already being best friends. All you need is to find the right partner, a woman with whom you click who is also interested in becoming fitter.

Your time together and your common goals should help your friendship deepen, naturally.

～ On Your Walks ～

During your walks, you will be helping your body become healthier. That's obvious. But the initial list of benefits—and perhaps the benefits you'll relish most—will come from your time with your friend. You will find that all you do is talk, talk, talk, and talk some more.

OUR TIME TO CHAT

We have always had so many things to talk over with each other. There have been so many times we've thought to ourselves, "I can't wait to tell her about this . . ."

If for some reason we didn't go for our walk, we still needed to chat. (But when did either of us have time for that once the day began and we belonged to everyone else?)

Even today, if for some reason we've missed a workout together, we seem to overflow with chatter the next time we see each other. It's as if we can't talk fast enough.

Just a few days ago, as we were getting ready to do sit-ups in our muscle-sculpting class, the instructor said to us (as we were immersed in conversation), "Maybe you two should just share one mat."

—Kim

While we didn't realize it then, we both needed this outlet because we were so busy with young kids, demanding careers and—oh yeah!—a husband and a marriage. It can be easy to sacrifice yourself to the demands of each day. The walks allowed us to find ourselves again. They enabled us to remember ourselves separately from all other things. Having that regular time to connect is what will boost your souls so that they can soar.

So what do we talk about? Chances are you won't have any problems coming up with topics. But here's a glimpse at what we have explored (and continue to explore!):

- Kids—Of course, if you're a mom it's virtually impossible not to talk about your kids. The beauty of sharing time with a friend at a similar phase in life means you will have a lot of common ground to cover, including birthday party ideas, schools, teachers, curriculum, homework, sports, commitments, friends, other parents, summer camps, sex education, religion, values, volunteering, activities, worries, fears, ages, and stages.
- Husbands—It's natural to want to vent on occasion, but don't turn your discussions into ongoing rag sessions about your husband or family. Negativity breeds more negativity. Instead, be positive. It will help you feel better throughout the rest of your day. If you need to vent, do it, get it over with, don't dwell, and move on to another topic.
- Work—Since we have always maintained our careers in rather creative ways—be it part-time, full-time, from home, or as consultants—juggling work commitments with our family priorities has always been an issue. We chat about projects, deadlines, struggles, goals, frustrations, bosses, and transitions. It has been helpful for us to be able to relate to the demands of balancing work and home, knowing that we both share the same values and priorities when it comes to our decisions and approaches.
- Details and To-Dos—Sometimes we find it useful to run through the list of what lies ahead for that day. It's a great time to organize ourselves and decide how to tackle that long, itemized list of to-dos.
- Schedules—In many ways, especially when our boys were attending the same preschool, we became second-string mommies for each other. We coordinated shared carpool schedules, playdates, and activities, and were able to step in to help each other whenever the need arose.
- Finds and Stumbles—One of our favorite topics has always been discussing new finds and information that we stumble upon. It may mean passing on an educational Web site for kids or giving

a recommendation for inexpensive manicures or detailing a great craft idea. We're always excited to give and to receive.

- Books—We are both avid readers and have similar taste in books. We've acted as a mini book club for two. We swap books and discuss what we've read. In the beginning of our walking routine, we continued to read our daily essays in *Simple Abundance* before we met each morning and then discussed our thoughts on it. That helped us think about aspects of our lives we hadn't thought about before. Ban Breathnach's ideas also prompted deeper discussions of spirituality, wants, goals, and needs.

- Interests and Passions—We chat about all the things in life we love and long for, including crafts, decorating ideas, vacation destinations, dreams, and even how we'll spend our retirement.

- Histories and Childhoods—We share our backgrounds. Sometimes that means discussing painful, often comical, and occasionally intimate, details from our childhoods and thoughts about our parents, college experiences, and past relationships.

- Praise and Kudos—Because we have became so intimately familiar with each others' schedules, commitments, interests, loves, passions, and pursuits, we are easily able to praise and applaud one another for our endeavors. The walks allowed us the opportunity to recognize each other's doing a great job. We also marveled at all we accomplished in a day—no one else could truly appreciate all that we were juggling and managing. And while plenty of women, moms, and wives juggle just as many commitments as we do, few ever receive praise for their efforts. Then and now, we give each other that much needed element of positive reinforcement.

∼ Developing Trust ∼

While it should go without saying, in order to foster a true sense of trust between you, there needs to be an unspoken rule that what is discussed on your walks is not fodder for gossip with other friends. Each of you needs to know that all secrets are safe, disclosures are protected, and privacy is paramount. You and your friend need to know that when you're ready to discuss something—in your own time—the other person will be there to listen and not to judge.

You also need to pay attention to one another when you're talking. Don't be inside your head thinking of the next thing you're going to say. Develop your listening skills. True, deep friendships blossom because the friends listen to one another, take turns, and respect each person's need to talk freely.

And, be sure to keep your promises. Being reliable and trustworthy is critical to allowing your friendship to become as deep as possible. Without trust, one or both will hold back. Yet creating an atmosphere of intimacy will allow each of you to work through life's daily issues and challenges. Talking through the bad times in your life and the obstacles you encounter is what will help you explore your options, determine strategies for tackling problems, and build emotional strength, resolve, and fortitude. The base of strength you find in your friendship will set you on solid ground when you're away from it.

Here are some final points that we believe are crucial for cultivating a deep, meaningful friendship:

- **Listen to and care about the other person.** Everyone wants to be heard, to know that her thoughts, her ideas, her stories matter. Showing that you care about the other person is as easy as taking the time to truly listen to her. By listening you'll learn. You'll learn about her childhood, college years, struggles, her most embarrassing moment, her marriage, dreams, regrets. The list is endless. The beauty of having a good friend in the here and now, is that you can be exactly who you are here and now. You don't have to feel stuck playing the role or wearing the persona you had when you were in grade school or college. In fact, you want to be certain that you are being as true to yourself as you can be—so that the friendship is built on honesty and integrity. In learning about your friend—the woman she is today—and in sharing your own stories and secrets, you'll be nurturing the friendship, helping it to become rich and full.
- **Be available for the other person, but respect her privacy and her family's privacy.** Remember, this is an adult relationship; you can't talk on the phone every night for hours as you might have

done with a childhood friend. Besides, who has the time for that? Plus, you do not want to create a situation in which your husband and children (or hers) feel threatened or neglected by the time you devote to the friendship. As you get to know each other better, be sure not to pry or become involved in her family matters or decisions. Only if your friend asks for your advice should you offer it. Most times, she may just need you to serve as a sounding board. So, be that. Be a great listener! Use your workout time to bond and have fun.

- **Get to know, understand, and respect your friend's moods.** We are all moody. Don't take it so personally if your friend is sullen or crabby. If your time together is quiet, that's okay (especially if you see each other daily.) You don't need to always fill the airtime with chatter.
- **And once again: never, ever share your private conversations with others.** Gossiping about your friend is a huge *no-no*. That's the quickest way to end your chance of ever getting close. Even if you never get *caught* gossiping, you'll always know you broke the bond. That alone will prevent you from getting as close as you possibly can.

∿ What If Your Friendship Doesn't Grow? ∿

Because you're on a new adventure together, you'll probably experience a honeymoon phase. You'll share ideas, idle chatter, and facts. You may progress to talking about your childhood, past loves, or exploits. You may entertain one another with funny stories and memories. After the honeymoon period ends, one of two things will happen: you'll continue to look forward to your time together, or . . . you won't.

If you find that the friendship starts to drain you of energy—leaving you feeling unhappier or more negative after your time together, you need to see that as a huge red flag. If that happens time after time, you may need to get out. The ultimate goal of this relationship is to leave you feeling uplifted, happy, lighter, more fulfilled and centered. Absolutely everyone should have a grown-up best friend, *but*, it needs to be the right person, the right friend. Life is too busy, time is too spare for you to spend it nurturing a relationship that doesn't deliver what you need. You can have a host of great friendships with women, but that does not necessarily mean any of them would work well as your best friend. If that's the case, you will need to have a candid, honest conversation to let your friend know that the arrangement isn't quite meeting your needs.

You may not find the friend who's right for you immediately, but you need to remain open to looking for her. Be patient and continue to look, but do not settle for something less than what you're looking for. You'll know when you have found that person.

If on the other hand, you look forward to every walk and your time together, then you can expect your friendship to start to take on a life of its own. Then, the power of the two of you working in tandem may allow you to attempt things you only dreamed of pursuing. You'll develop a confidence brought on by having a cheerleader in your corner. As you and your friend begin to listen to what's in your souls—the whispers of your dreams—you'll start believing in each other's ability to pursue them. That's when the friendship has the power to change your life.

∾ How to Address a Problem or ∾ Confront an Issue

This is an interesting one for us to give advice on. Neither one of us confronts issues or problems readily. We've come to believe that most problems and issues are generally not worth addressing. So, if you get wound tight over small issues, try to roll with things a bit more. Try not to take things so personally. As you continue to pursue fitness and as your confidence grows, you may notice that fewer things bother or upset you. But if you do decide to address a problem or issue, wait at least a day or two first before you bring it up. That will help you avoid reacting to something when you are mad or feeling emotional. If you do decide to address a problem, be prepared to bring forth a possible solution and to talk it through. Also be prepared to accept an apology and be done with it. Everyone makes mistakes. That alone should not be a reason to toss a good friend. If you truly find that the issue or problem cannot be resolved, then it may be time to move on. Again there is much peace and power to be found with the right friend—be willing to do the work to find her. In the end, you'll both be glad you did.

❧ **Notes** ❧

If you ever need to gather your thoughts regarding a tough issue you want to address with your friend use this space to help you form your ideas and points.

_____

_____

_____

_____

_____

_____

❧ **Notes** ❧

If you need to search for another partner, think back to some of your older, dearer friends. Think of the qualities they possess. Write those qualities down. Now think of women you know who resemble them in manner or personality or style. Write down their names. Perhaps one of these women might be a great potential partner for you.

_____

_____

_____

_____

_____

_____

CHAPTER 4

JOINING A GYM

ONCE YOU'VE BEEN in your routine for quite a while, you will have achieved an important milestone: taking better care of yourself. The longer you continue on that path, the greater the chance that you'll continue in that direction. However, there may be times when you start to feel bored with your routine. Don't be fooled into thinking that your restlessness means that you're bored with exercise. Don't use your boredom as an excuse to quit. Instead, think back to how far you've come. Remember how difficult it is to start a routine from scratch. Do you really want to forsake all your hard work up until this point? Start to see boredom as a sign that you're simply ready for a new challenge—perhaps you are ready to join a gym or to try a different activity altogether.

Other events may also prompt a need for change. You may face an illness or an injury that may cause you to reassess your entire approach to fitness. That's how it happened for us. When we first decided to change our walking routine, it wasn't because we were bored or restless. At the time, we were completely content with our routine and our accomplishments. But by 2000, things began to change.

∽ Kris Looks Back ∽

You may reach a point in your life when you realize that your body is aging and you are not quite the same as you use to be. That moment came for me at the age of thirty-five when I was told that I had to have surgery, involving an incision across my stomach. My recovery was difficult. I had no upper-arm or upper-body strength to push myself up out of bed. It was frightening to be so reliant on other people for even my most basic needs. It was a stunning realization: I had not taken good enough care of my body. I vowed that I would prepare myself better, in case I should ever face surgery again.

After my recovery, my husband suggested that I make better use of our morning walk time, since I was already getting up and in a routine (he never understood the whole "chitchat" thing.) I talked with Kim about it, but pretty much announced that I would be giving up our walking time so that I could start a training program at the gym (which my husband had joined a year earlier, although I had never gone). Once again, I was resorting to old patterns and habits, where I plunged myself into an exercise plan as a quick and rash response to solving a problem with my body. In the past, it had often been in response to gaining a few pounds. This time it was in an effort to correct the mounting health problems I was facing. Initially, my focus was to increase my arm strength. I wanted to be able to push myself up and out of bed with my arms and not have to rely on my stomach muscles. I knew I needed to take the next step. But it never dawned on me that I might be on the verge of making a critical error by forsaking the partnership we'd built and trying to go it alone (which, of course, had never worked as a long-term solution for me before). With hindsight, I know that I never would have been successful without my friend going along with it.

∽ Kim Looks Back ∽

I panicked when Kris announced that she was going to join a gym. I was so addicted to our walks and our time together, that I didn't want it to end. I also feared that convincing my husband to shell out the cash for a gym membership was going to be an uphill battle. He had seen me waste money on gym memberships before. Yet for the first time, I had the confidence in myself that I could and would follow through and use the membership. He wasn't so sure. As I argued my points, I tried to emphasize to him that this time would be different because we were already in a routine. We had proven ourselves and our ability to stick to a workout. This time, we would simply go to the gym instead of walking, using the same time slot we had already secured each day. In the end, it took some all-out begging to get him to acquiesce. The burden was clearly on me to prove that I could stick to it. Failure would mean a lifetime of well-deserved "I told you so's." By the time he gave me the OK, Kris had already been going to the gym for two weeks by herself. That gave us a taste of what it would be like going it alone without each other. Neither one of us was jazzed about that prospect. I knew there was no way I would continue to walk, as long as I had to do it alone. I also knew there was no way that I would join a gym, on my own, if she hadn't joined it first.

After signing my membership papers, one of the very first things I did was have a health assessment. The personal trainer, Mark, had already given Kris her assessment and worked up a plan for her, which included the Nautilus equipment and some aerobic/cardio work. Because he knew we were going to be working out together, he created a plan for me that mirrored hers. That way, we could be on the same program. He introduced me to all of the machines and to the proper technique. Then he wished me good luck.

◇ Walking, Talking, and Weights ◇

We enjoyed our walks so much that when we headed inside to the gym, we simply maintained our walking routine using the treadmills and elliptical machines. We used the Nautilus equipment, alternating between focusing on arms and abs one day and legs the next. This covered our routine for the week.

Our inside workouts resembled our neighborhood walks, where we chatted and strolled. That was our cardio plan. As intimidated and awed as we were by the gym regulars and their workout routines, we certainly weren't going to jump in feet first and do anything too taxing or strenuous. We didn't care to compete with them. In fact, we barely broke a sweat each day. That didn't matter to us, because we were still proud to be doing something consistently, every morning of every weekday.

Even today, we believe that's a tremendous accomplishment and is a perfectly reasonable approach to becoming fit. If that's your philosophy too, keep at it. Again, you're still doing something. You're doing more than you were doing before you picked up this book. We don't believe there's any need or reason to rush into change or to accelerate your intensity until you're ready. We have always taken slow, small steps toward progress. And in time toward big results. It works. When the time is right to try something new or to adjust your intensity, then you'll know it. If that day never comes, yet you continue walking and perhaps lifting light weights (and of course, getting a regular dose of friendship), then everything you're doing is leading you to greater fitness. That's what matters most.

∼ Are You Ready for a Change? ∼

Other than having an epiphany and thinking to yourself, "I'm ready for a change!" it might be hard to recognize the signs that you're ready to try something different. As we mentioned, often the first sign is a sense of boredom. It's a ho-hum feeling about going for your walk or your workout. It's natural to have occasional days or stretches of time when you feel that way, but if that feeling lingers, it might be time to consider adding some variety to your routine. Another sign that boredom is settling in is when you or your partner start to skip your workout days. If you start to see these patterns, chat about them. Maybe it's the right time to take it up a notch and to challenge yourselves a bit more.

When you're in it together, you come to rely on the benefits of your time and exercise. That is the beauty and the strength of the friendship bond, and that's when you realize its power. If one of you gets motivated to take it to the next level (after your core routine is established), the other one is not likely to be left behind.

That is what we've discovered in working as a team. We help each other become better. We challenge each other to take it to the next level, and not just in the arena of exercise. We also support each other as we raise the bar. That element of pushing each other cannot be underestimated. It's the concept of friendly, healthy competition that can spur you on to "greatness"—or at least to lift one more set, to run one more mile, or to get up early yet again.

So, if one of you is contemplating joining a gym, use your walks to talk through the pros and the cons, to pinpoint how you might make it work, to discuss what the new routine might look like, and to evaluate what your goals might be. Remember, it's in your best interest to arrive at decisions as a team. That's the only way that you'll be able to keep the power of the friendship working for you. It's also the only way you can maintain the integrity of your time together.

In the end, it doesn't really matter whose idea it is. What matters is that you're both behind it. If you are hesitant to make a big change to your routine but your partner wants to proceed, then you may need to take a leap of faith and trust that your partner is in a position to lead you down the right road. After all, you can do greater work together than you can apart.

∾ Joining a Gym ∾

Joining a gym is just one option. But it's a relatively common approach. Here are some tips to get you started on your research and on making decisions that will meet both of your needs.

- **Set a monthly budget for your membership costs.** Develop a budget that is reasonable and workable for both of you. If one of you can afford a more costly gym, then you need to compromise, so that both of you can find a gym that meets your needs but doesn't blow your budget.

  As you research the costs in your area and compare pricing, be sure to investigate whether or not the club offers half-day versus full-day memberships or if they offer month-to-month plans as opposed to an annual fee.

- **Check out the hours.** This is especially important if maintaining your routine requires you to get together in the wee hours of the morning or late at night. Many gyms these days are open twenty-four hours a day. Most open early, before the crack of dawn and stay open fairly late. Be sure the ones you consider meet your needs. Don't kid yourself into thinking you'll try a new time and establish a new routine. Instead, fold the gym time into the time and routine you've already established. That will ensure success.

- **When looking at locations, go for convenience.** It's likely a host of gyms are nearby. As you research them, choose only those that are within a ten-minute drive of your homes (or offices). If it takes more than ten minutes to get there, it's too far.
- **Get some guest passes.** Many gyms offer free guest passes as an incentive to get potential members to join. Don't be afraid to ask for passes, so that you can get a feel for the facility. Be sure to visit it during the hours you will use it. This will help you gauge whether or not it's crowded at that time (which may be a factor in how long it takes you to work out).
- **Head for the showers.** If you will be using the shower or changing facility, be sure to check them out before you join! Look to see how clean it is and whether it's in disrepair—does it boast mold or peeling paint? Do the showers have curtains or doors? All of this will have an effect on how comfortable you feel while you're there.
- **Tour the entire facility.** You may not be interested in swimming, but be sure to walk through the pool area if there is one. Tour the entire facility to check out all of the equipment it offers. After all, you never know when you may want to vary your routine, change your activity, or try something new.
- **Grab a flyer for class schedules.** Classes are a great way to add variety and to try something new, with little risk and commitment. Review the class schedule so you'll know which options fit with your regular workout time. Discuss which types of classes you may both be interested in trying.
- **Investigate the ancillary services.** It's important to find out what other types of services the club offers, such as babysitting. Also find out if there are additional costs for these services and what hours they are offered.
- **Find out if there are any family-oriented activities that take place on weekends.** Some facilities cater to families on the weekends. They may host youth swimming or basketball programs. Find out if there are options for your kids, if and when you both need to squeeze in some time together on a weekend while the kids are home. These are great "Plan B" options for times when you've missed a workout because you were sick or because your husband

had to travel or you had to attend an early morning meeting. (Of course, if you don't have kids, you may want to know this as well, so you can plan your schedules around *avoiding* peak kid time!)

∽ Scheduling an Assessment ∽

When you first join the gym, you may want to consider signing up for a health assessment. Usually this involves meeting with a certified personal trainer. He or she will likely weigh you, do a body-fat test, measure your anaerobic capacity and your heart rate, count how many sit-ups you can do in one minute, and test your flexibility. On the one hand, you can use the information as a baseline to track your progress. On the other hand, it may deliver some rather depressing statistics. Whether or not you choose to do it together is a personal, private matter and is a decision you should make on your own. When we did ours we did them separately and never shared the results with each other.

One benefit of a health assessment is that after all of the torturous tests and measurements the personal trainer will give you a tour of the gym, introduce you to all of the machines and services, and create a workout routine for you to follow. Even having the trainer introduce you to the gym requires courage. But it's worth it. You do not want to try to figure out the machines by yourself. You also do not want to "create" your own workout, since you may risk injury if you are not using proper technique. With a plan from the personal trainer, you have a starting point and a way to measure progress. Otherwise, you're at the mercy of which machine looks less threatening on any given day. Plus, the plan should give you a well-rounded approach to exercise because trainers usually try to address every aspect of your fitness—from cardio to strength.

∽ What Do You Do Once You Get There? ∽

Even with your exercise plan in hand, your first days at the gym can feel awkward and intimidating. Because we had a slight gap of time between when we began going together, we did not get the chance to give each other support during our initial visits. Yet that was certainly one of the times that relying on our friendship would have helped us both. Be sure to venture forth together, if at all possible.

Fighting the Intimidation Factor

The idea of going to a gym is very different from strolling around the neighborhood. There are machines to contend with, rooms and rooms of weights, crowded exercise classes, and issues of workout etiquette (such as, don't wear perfume!) to consider. While the initial tour of a gym—its clanking, whirring background sounds and shiny, sleek look—can be inspiring and exciting, the first few times you attend may have you trembling with fear.

Perhaps the biggest problem is battling your own self-consciousness. It's easy to think that everyone is looking at you or noticing that you're new to the club. In some cases that might be true. For us, it definitely was. Since we go so early in the morning, the only people who are there are those who are committed to working hard on their fitness. Five thirty in the morning is not the time for the casual exerciser to drop in and give a workout a try. We probably stuck out as the new kids on the block even more than we realized.

Because you might feel as if all eyes are on you, it's easy to think: *I'll start going to the gym when I look better in leggings.* Or, *I'll start after I lose some weight.* That's not the right approach. If you and your friend have decided to give the gym a try, then go for it! Don't hold yourself back. What you don't realize today, is that even the most intensely committed gym rats will gain tremendous respect for you if you simply continue to show up, each and every day, day after day. They're not scrutinizing what you wear or what you look like or how much you weigh. They scrutinize your work ethic. They will notice how consistently you attend. They will notice when you don't show up. So don't be afraid of what anyone thinks of you while you're there at the gym; it's what they think of you when you're not there that is really telling.

For example, there are two women who have been regularly attending our Wednesday kickboxing class. This class is by far one of the most challenging workouts we do. We're impressed when we see them (since they are a bit overweight) attend the class week after week. We still remember how painfully sore we were after each class when we first started. It hurt to squat down to go to the bathroom. It hurt while we tried to sleep at night. It hurt as we hobbled to our cars stiff-legged to drive the kids to school. Even now, if we take a week or two off (because of vacation or illness), we know we will be greeted by intense soreness when we return. As a class, we suspect it's even harder for them because it's such a demanding, physical workout. Each and every one of us who regularly attends the class understands what a tremendous accomplishment it is to simply endure and then to return the following week. The mere fact that they have come back again and again, despite the soreness, despite the intense challenge, speaks volumes about what they are capable of accomplishing. They just may not realize it yet! And frankly, we have no idea if they've lost weight, if they see changes in their body, or if they feel good about themselves. We only know that we hope they keep coming back and we respect them more and more each time they walk through the door. There's no doubt that if they continue to show up and work hard, they will experience benefits and results. If for some reason they stopped coming, it would seem a shame that all that hard work and achievement was abandoned.

Find Your Role Model

During your first weeks, take a look around at the regulars in the club—the gym rats. You can't help but notice them. Consider picking one or two to model yourself after. Take note of what they are doing, quietly following behind them or in their footsteps to see what their workout looks like. Don't do their workout (because they'll be at a different level than you are), but use them for inspiration to get to the gym each day.

Our first role model was a woman named Annie. She is by far the most physically fit woman we have ever personally known. And because she is older than us, it seems even more impressive (it's not that big a deal to see a young, fit person. After all, that's what you'd expect to see). Annie's a machine. Her muscles ripple out from her back and shoulders. Her biceps bulge. She runs fast. She can do endless push-ups, jumping jacks, and squats. She swims. She cycles. She is highly competitive. And she's a tiny, pixie of a woman, weighing no more than one hundred pounds. We've never aspired to become Annie. We'll never even come close to accomplishing what she can. Yet she's tremendously inspirational, particularly in terms of her work ethic. "Did you see how many push-ups she did?" we'd squawk after a muscle-sculpting class. Or, "Oh my gosh, did you see how fast she was running?" It might seem easy to get discouraged having an Annie around. Quite the contrary. Standing next to her in a class, can push us to work just a bit harder. Each time we work a bit harder, our fitness level improves. Month after month, and then year after year, it's those tiny daily improvements that make all the difference in the world.

In time, if you can start to say that you see the same faces over and over again, and be able to recite their specific workout routine and work ethic, then you will notice that you are becoming one of them. How does that happen? Because being intimately aware of the gym rats, their names, and their routines, means you have been consistent in going to the gym. Consistency delivers results—in mind, body, and spirit. How do we know? Because ironically, some people (like the two women in our kickboxing class) might now perceive us as gym rats. Over time, and without even noticing it, you can be transformed by your time in the gym when you go routinely. Clearly, it wasn't all that long ago that we remember the challenge of walking through the doors and entering a whole new, intimidating world. Don't let your fear of that world prevent you from joining it.

∽ Notes ∽

As you scout around and conduct research on which health clubs are right for you, use this space to take notes on your findings.

_____

_____

_____

_____

_____

_____

_____

_____

CHAPTER 5

TRYING SOMETHING NEW

I F YOU'VE BEEN GOING to the gym regularly or have been in your walking routine for a while, you might—once again—be ready to try something new. That "something new" might encompass a different activity, class, or exercise. The beauty of trying something new with a friend, is that you're *together*. It's far easier to break out of a rut when you have someone to do it with. It's also far easier to put yourself "out there," to be vulnerable, when you don't feel completely alone. As you contemplate trying something new, vary your exercise rather than your actual routine (the time and days that you get together). When you stray too far from what's been successful for you, you risk getting off track. However, there's no guarantee that all forays into new arenas will turn out well (but you're always better for having tried). This chapter explores a range of options available to you and how you can view each one you try as an adventure.

∼ Kim Looks Back ∼

Several years ago, we decided to give yoga a try. Kris had seen the one-night-a-week class offered at our local rec center. We decided to supplement our walking routine with yoga. We registered for the same class, but I was unable to attend the first couple of sessions. She went on her own, and seemed to enjoy it. She found it relaxing and told me about various aspects of the class, such as the instructor's use of bells during certain moves. By the third class, we were able to go together.

After a few poses, he started to correct Kris's postures. He'd move her arm or her leg to place it in a certain spot. But he wasn't really correcting the other students in quite the same, hands-on way. Every time he corrected her, he said her formal name, Kristine, in this long, deep guttural whisper. It was creepy and also comical (since I knew no one other than her mom ever called her Kristine, and she hates being called Kristine. It made me chuckle each time I heard him say it).

At one point, we had our butts pushed up against the wall, with our legs high in the air spread out to each side. I felt so vulnerable in that pose, but I knew Kris had to be dying, especially as he continued to whisper "Kristine . . . Kristine" as he corrected her position.

Then he decided he was going to demonstrate a "new" move for the night. He began a long explanation of the origins of this move, talking about how he was going to return us to the days when we experienced pure innocence—as infants. Because he had a thick accent, it was rather difficult to understand all that he was saying. We kept looking at each other, wondering, "Did he really just say that he was going to have us feel it 'deep in our pleasure zone'?"

Then he started to demonstrate the move. He curled up into a fetal position and began to writhe on the floor. As he did, he rolled and turned and twisted and contorted. He continued on for several minutes. As I watched, I was becoming painfully, embarrassingly aware that he actually seemed to be climaxing right in front of our eyes.

I looked around the room to see if anyone else was as shocked and horrified as I was. But I couldn't look at Kris, because I was afraid I'd burst out laughing right there and then.

Once he was done and his writhing, twisting, and contorting stopped, he stood up and turned out the lights. As he did, he said, "Now it's your turn."

I thought, "There is no way I would do that 'move' in front of Harry (my husband), in the privacy of our own bedroom, let alone in here!"

It was pitch black in the room. Of course, I was too wimpy to make a scene and flee. So, I balled up onto my mat, facedown, with my eyes tightly shut. I could hear the swishing sound of other bodies moving.

Every once in a while I would flex my arm or throw out my hand. I'd open one eye to try to see what other people were doing. That's when I noticed that the guy next to Kris was actually getting into the activity. He was rolling and having spasms all over his mat. He seemed to be having as much fun with it as the instructor had. I couldn't wait until the lights came back on and we could go home.

Once the class ended, I couldn't even look over where Kris was sitting. When we started to walk out of the class, all I could whisper as we raced to the car was, "Don't say anything!" As soon as we jumped in, we burst out laughing, shrieking until our stomachs hurt and tears filled our eyes. That night, we struggled to retell the story to our husbands because we kept laughing so hard.

For months after that class, if I met someone who said they enjoyed yoga, I'd interrogate them. I'd describe our experience and ask, "Is that what yoga is really like?" I couldn't imagine what the craze was all about. Each time I told someone our story, she'd look at me oddly. "No," she'd shake her head, "I haven't done that move before." Yet she'd never outright say, "That's not at all what yoga is like." As a result, it was difficult to distinguish between whether it was yoga we didn't care for or simply the instructor and his approach. It was an eternity before we were willing to give yoga another try.

∼ Kris Looks Back ∼

We had been regulars at the gym for quite a while. Each morning as we strolled on the treadmill, a group of people, mostly men, were cycling across from us. One of them was named Don. He was an instructor who taught kickboxing and muscle-sculpting classes. He had a hardy, boisterous laugh that echoed throughout the gym. He knew everyone in the gym and everyone seemed to gravitate toward him.

Often as we were leaving, he'd shout over to us, "You need to come try one of my classes." We'd giggle, blush, and stammer some lame excuse. I knew there was no way I was going to take one of his classes.

As we'd leave the gym on the days when he taught classes, we'd strain to catch a glimpse of what was going on behind the glass walls. Given our yoga class experience, we weren't going to jump headfirst into anything we weren't completely comfortable with. As we watched, we couldn't imagine keeping up with the students in the class, let alone him. We'd been getting a lot of ribbing from him about our slow-paced walks. I certainly wasn't going to embarrass myself in one of his classes in front of his whole crew.

It's hard to remember how we eventually got the courage to give it a try. Perhaps, because he was such a powerful presence in the gym—a gregarious extrovert—it was difficult to ignore his banter and invitations. Our consistency in going to the gym was paying off in added confidence. We'd gained enough so that we were at least willing to test the waters. Yet walking in that very first day to his kickboxing class we were anxious and intimidated.

He made us feel welcome as did all the students in the class, who had seen us on the treadmills strolling and yakking for months. It was a brutal class. We must've done hundreds of jumping jacks, followed by at least one hundred lunges, leg lifts, and push-ups. Our calves burned. Our chests hurt. Once the class was over, we could barely lift our arms to our ears. It was a challenge just putting the key in the ignition to drive home. But we couldn't wait to go back. We had thoroughly enjoyed ourselves. We left that first class feeling challenged, energized, rejuvenated, whipped, tired, and happy, even though we struggled through much of it.

Then the next day came. We couldn't even walk, let alone lower ourselves onto the commode to pee. Just standing up once we were sitting down was a challenge. Our walk became a shuffle, because it hurt to lift our legs high enough to take a step. Curbs would make us cringe. Still, we couldn't wait to return the following Wednesday.

It's amazing how one experience can have a tremendous impact on how you feel about an exercise, activity, or class. We didn't try yoga again for another two years after our first experience. Yet, we've attended every single Wednesday kickboxing class that Don has taught for the past four years (unless we were sick or on vacation). Eventually, in the privacy of our own homes, in front of the VCR, we gave yoga another shot. Thankfully we did, because it's one of our favorite activities and is a terrific complement to running.

What we've learned is that as you try new activities, you'll have good experiences and not-so-good ones. Don't give up on an activity prematurely. Give it a few tries, with different instructors or trainers, in different environments, before you decide whether or not it's right for you.

Even though we've been fairly adventurous in trying new things over the last few years, we have only scratched the surface in terms of the options available. For as many as we've tried (cycling, running, yoga, Pilates), there are twice as many that we haven't (swimming, rowing, team sports, and more). Here's what we've tried and here's what we've found over many trials and errors, as we've searched for variety. (For specific details on how to perform certain exercises or how to approach a certain activity, please refer to appendix B, "Posture and Activity Tips and Techniques.")

∼ Taking a Class ∼

Classes are offered everywhere, from gyms to local rec centers. To help ensure finding a good class with a great instructor, talk to people you know. Ask them for their recommendations, particularly of the instructors. If you're at a gym and you're too shy to ask, then simply observe which classes seem to be most crowded and which ones the gym regulars attend. Those will be the classes that are superior to others.

There are a host of reasons to consider taking a class. And there are more types of classes than you can imagine, from traditional aerobics and step classes to cycling/spinning, yoga, Pilates, dancing, muscle sculpting, kickboxing, core strength training, and so on. Plus, there are always new classes, crazes, and equipment innovations to keep the options growing.

Classes are ideal because they:

- offer a range of options from which to choose, so there's bound to be one that will appeal to you.
- allow you and your friend to enjoy the same activity even if you're at different levels (for example, maybe you can do more push-ups than your friend can, but you can still both enjoy the same muscle sculpting class).
- deliver variety even within the class (rarely does an instructor do the exact same moves and routines week after week).
- work several muscle groups at one time.
- can push you beyond where you would push yourself.
- can cure boredom.
- require little long-term commitment.

The downside of taking a class is that it can be intimidating. That's one of the key reasons to do it with your friend. Sure, you may feel silly, weak, uncoordinated, winded, and even frustrated at first. But your adventures will always provide great fodder for the ride home. Classes can also be difficult to work into your specific routine. Yet finding a class with an instructor you thoroughly enjoy, is well worth the search. So keep your eyes open and scout out the best options for you both. Make sure, however, that you always provide opportunities for the two of you to connect regularly, to attend together, and to maintain your routine. Try as often as possible to drive together to the class or to give yourselves time to warm up with a walk on the treadmill before the class begins. If the classes don't support your ability to do that, it might be better for the partnership to pursue other activities (or to only take classes once a week or so).

Aerobics, Kickboxing, Step Classes

At some point in your life, you've probably taken one form or another of an aerobics, step, jazzercise, or kickboxing class. There are high- and low-impact options from which to choose. Each offers something a little different and each instructor's choreography will vary. It's a personal preference.

- Aerobics classes can range from the traditional (grapevine) to the funkier, hip-hop type of dance classes. If you're not certain which one is better for you, try to observe a class before you plunge ahead. And always look for the beginner's level when trying something new.
- Step classes can also be wide ranging. Some are basic with instructors who call out a handful of simple moves. Others can be highly complex, choreographed routines that take weeks and months to master. Again, start at square one at the entry level. You can always advance to another level, but taking a class that exceeds your abilities is a great way to get hurt.
- Kickboxing can vary from a class that offers punches and kicks at a moderate pace to highly intense sports-conditioning classes.

Cycle/Spinning Classes

Cycle and "spinning" classes involve stationary bikes, pulsing music, and an instructor to direct speed and cadence. These classes are popular with different types of people and athletes. Usually, mostly women take aerobics or step classes. However, a good cycling and spinning class can draw the competitive triathletes, cyclists, and runners, as well as all others in the gym. Thus, it can be the most intimidating class to join for the first time but also very inspiring.

Muscle-Sculpting Classes

Muscle-sculpting classes involve some form of resistance or weight training, and offer a nice break from high-impact, hard cardio workouts. They're also a good complement to other types of workouts. Muscle-sculpting classes can introduce you to a variety of different weight- or strength-training techniques, including:

- hand weights (dumbbells) and bars
- squats
- push-ups
- stability balls
- bands and jump ropes

Yoga and Pilates

Yoga and Pilates classes offer so many options and benefits with a variety of types to choose from. Yoga classes usually focus on breathing, calming the mind, stretching, and lengthening the body through a variety of poses. Pilates (named after its creator Joseph Pilates) focuses on these as well, but also emphasizes strengthening the core (or trunk) of the body through a series of deliberate, controlled movements. Yoga is an ideal complement to running. Many of its positions, such as the "down dog" and the "pigeon," are perfect stretches that can help runners avoid injury. Both can help improve your posture and leave you feeling relaxed, centered, and more mindful of your body.

If you are new to yoga, find a "live" class that you like before you try yoga on video or TV. With an instructor, you should get hands-on correction of your form and posture. Sometimes they will actually move you into the proper positioning. This helps you know the "feel" of a position so that you will be able to self-correct as you improve. (If your instructor does not correct your poses or offer the class "cues" on form and posture, you should find another instructor.) That one-on-one mentoring is crucial to fully enjoying and benefiting from either yoga or Pilates.

While in a yoga or Pilates class, do what your body can do comfortably. While you want to challenge yourself, you don't want to push yourself beyond your limits (and risk injury). It's easy to think that since the positions are subtle and controlled, you should "intensify" them in some way by pushing harder or forcing something unnaturally. Instead, listen to the instructor, follow her cues, and try to be mindful of the movements you are making and the position of your body. Doing any movement in yoga or Pilates can be challenging, if you are truly controlling the movement of your body properly.

Lifting Weights

Lifting weights can prompt quick changes in your body, particularly in your arms (biceps, triceps, and back). But it's important that you utilize proper technique and maintain proper posture when doing so. If you have joined a gym, you should have an assessment by a certified personal trainer and have her design a program for you and your friend together. If the trainer knows you are going to be workout partners, she can design a program to meet both of your needs and goals. This way, you can support each other, hang out together, chitchat, and progress on the same path. In addition, the trainer will introduce you to the machines and equipment, as well as demonstrate proper form and technique. If you are new to weight training, using a trainer is a much better approach to starting out, than simply trying to read about proper form in a book, magazine, or on the Internet.

At the gym, you will need to decide whether or not you want your program to incorporate the circuit weight-training machines or the free weights (dumbbells, barbells, and weight benches). Usually, the circuit machines are located in a slightly different area than the free weights. Because the serious weight lifters are found in the free-weight room, it can be less intimidating to start out using the circuit machines. Once you build up a base of strength using the circuit—and some more confidence—consider having your personal trainer introduce you to the free weights. That way you'll have more options and a well-rounded approach. Plus, with free-weight experience you can do your workout outside of the gym, while at home or on the road if you want.

Running

As an aerobic activity, running burns more calories than any other single activity. Yet, people usually either love running or hate it. Nonrunners complain that running hurts their knees or that they're simply not the running type. We can relate. Neither one of us ever considered ourselves the running types. But over the last several years, running has literally changed our lives.

The key to experiencing success when you try to run, is to not go too far, too fast. Most people venture out and try to run a mile or more their very first day. Then they follow that up with several more days of the same schedule. Or, they try to go out and run too fast, without understanding issues of pacing and rhythm. All of which can lead to a host of problems, from feelings of discouragement and frustration to serious injury.

If you're interested in starting to run, you need to start slowly in order to build up your distance, your stamina, your strength. This is especially important for those who may have once been runners. Just because you used to be able to run five miles in college does not mean your body can perform or adapt as it once did. Start at square one and work your way up in small increments, allowing yourself time to acclimate to running.

Running Together

When you and your friend run together, you can take a couple different approaches:

- You can run together at the same pace. If you can talk comfortably while you run, then you're at the right pace for a beginner's running program. Chatting is a good self-check to ensure you're not going too fast, too soon.

- You can start off together and then separate, going at your own individual pace. If you don't really like running with someone or you're not comfortable doing so, you can do your warm-up walk and stretching session together, then head off independently. You'll want to follow the same route though. If you do, usually you'll find that you're within eyesight of one another, just not in lockstep.

There is no right or wrong way. Just do what feels comfortable for you both.

As you can see, there are endless options. We've only touched upon a few of the most common ones available. Look at any foray into new arenas as an adventure. After all, at a bare minimum, you may walk away with your own funny yoga story to keep you howling for years to come.

CHAPTER 6

INJURIES AND
INTERRUPTIONS

E HAVE ALL experienced an interruption or a hiccup in our best-laid plans. You may have arranged a great beach vacation with friends and family only for it to be canceled because of a hurricane. Or, perhaps you worked months on a deadline, only to lose all of your work when your PC crashed. Your pursuit of fitness is no different from the rest of your life. It's not immune. You can expect at some point, you will have to deal with an interruption or injury. But, we have found that you can discover a silver lining to the clouds. Every injury and interruption we have experienced has in some way furthered our commitment and determination to pursue getting and staying fit.

∼ Kris Looks Back ∼

It was late June, and Kim and I were vacationing together with our families at the Outer Banks in North Carolina. I knew that following the vacation, I was scheduled to repeat the exact same surgery I had just fully recovered from only six months earlier. I had so many emotions I was dealing with—intense fear, a deep sadness, plus aching disappointment. I was terrified of the surgery itself, based on the difficult recovery I had just experienced. I was deeply saddened to know that I was moving farther away from being able to have more children. And I ached with disappointment to know that all the progress I had made with my health in the months since the first surgery appeared to be a waste—I'd be forced to begin all over again.

Looking back at the two surgeries, I now see that they served as opportunities for us. Each of them caused us to reevaluate our fitness routines and to make some modifications. At the time of the first surgery in January 2000, we were still in our walking routine. However, during my recovery, I did not walk and neither did Kim. My recovery was difficult. While in the hospital, I was completely reliant on the nursing staff for all of my needs. That prompted me to decide to join a gym, which Kim joined too.

Six months later, I faced the same surgery. But, two things differed from that first experience. First, my recovery was much easier. It was hard to believe that in just a few months of lifting weights at the gym, I was so much stronger and better prepared for the surgery and recovery process. In the hospital I could actually lift myself out of bed almost immediately after the surgery. This was a huge revelation for me: that concrete, tangible fitness gains can be made in a relatively short amount of time.

The second difference between the first surgery and the second was that Kim continued our exercise routine while I was laid up. Within six weeks of the surgery, I was allowed to return to the gym. While Kim had not progressed our routine, she had maintained it. And I was anxious to return. I did, however, need to modify some of the exercises to accommodate my weakened abdominal muscles. Because we had been doing a moderate cardio workout and weight training, I simply adjusted my approach to some of the exercises. For the most part, I was able to jump right back in and work even harder to make up for lost time.

I experienced another interruption to our routine in September 2001, when I had a miscarriage. Prior to the pregnancy, Kim and I were running and attending Don's kickboxing class faithfully. As soon as I knew I was pregnant, I modified my workouts to be lower in intensity and impact. I had finally become pregnant after seven long years. Moreover, the pregnancy had occurred without any assistance from doctors—just the help of my husband. I wondered if my regular doses of physical activity and improved fitness level helped. I was filled with happiness, but it was quickly lost when only eight weeks later I found out that my identical twin girls were gone. I mourned the loss for a long time. Even still today, when I see children, a bittersweet smile can cross my face.

Within days after the loss of the babies, I turned to exercise to heal me and I returned to our routine harder than ever. We began running more. As we did, we both wore headsets. We seemed to need the music as motivation for accomplishing our longer, faster runs. I wonder now though, if I also needed that added time and space to heal. And if so, did Kim intuitively allow me that time and space? Whatever the reasons we turned to music when we ran as opposed to turning to our traditional chats, it gave me the chance to allow small pieces of emotions to spill forward slowly so that I could deal with them as best I could. Over months and months of logging in miles and as my heart was slowly healing, we were both becoming "runners." That phase of our journey sparked our passion for running. Once again, one of life's interruptions served to further advance our fitness pursuits. Moreover, it was evidence that exercise can be used not only to make you healthier so you can avoid such issues, but it can be used as a powerful coping tool in times of crisis and despair. Exercise can be the one piece of the puzzle that helps you hold it together, when you feel as if the rest of your life is falling apart. While I can only speculate, it's frightening for me to imagine how my days, my marriage, my ability to be a good mommy, might have been affected had I not been able to turn to exercise and the calming ways of our routine.

∾ Kim Looks Back ∾

I don't have to look too far back to be reminded of an injury or an interruption. In fact, according to my watch it's probably time to put some more ice on my quad muscle. I've been nursing a slight pull or strain in my left quad since last Monday. At first, it was a teeny, tiny little twinge of an injury. I felt it during one of our short four-mile runs, a slight sensation that stretched up the front of my leg. By that afternoon, it felt pretty sore and was tender when I walked.

Next week, our training plan calls for us to run twenty miles in preparation for the Marine Corps Marathon. Running twenty miles with a teeny, tiny little twinge seems like a sure way to create one big, ugly injury. So, I've been babying it, trying to nurse it back to health. I've iced it and taken Advil round the clock. All I can think of each time I move or walk is, "Do I feel it? Does this hurt? How about when I do this?"

By Friday, it seemed to be getting better. And then I tripped over the dog and landed full force on my left foot. That really strained it. Quickly, I've progressed from concern to fear to a mix of outright terror and melancholy. How long is it going to take to get better? What if I think it's better, but it's not, and I hurt it worse? What if my training gets derailed, how will I recover? What if it doesn't get better? How long can I go without running on it, before I start to lose the endurance, strength, and mental fortitude I've gained so far? Will I have to run my next long run beneath a shadow of fear that I'll injure it worse? And what if it goes out on me while I'm ten miles from home, then what will I do? Will Kris continue on with our training plan and push past me and my capabilities?

It's all so overwhelming. A huge part of my life revolves around not just a workout routine but a training plan, and around my health. Does the slightest injury have the power to derail all of that? The key for me is to figure out how to bridge the gaps between healing the injury, addressing the need for rest, and still moving toward the goal. So, several times throughout the day I recalculate my plan, scrutinizing the number of weeks between now and the race, trying to focus on how and when I can wisely get back to my routine and to feeling healthy.

Of course, it wasn't always this way. There was a time when having an itchy-ouchy meant I could sleep in. I could relax and skip a workout without feeling guilty.

That frame of mind began to shift a bit when Kris had her second surgery. By then, we were already working out in the gym. While she needed to take some time to have the surgery and to recover, there was no doubt that she wanted to return to our normal routine as quickly as possible.

I felt a huge sense of responsibility to keep the routine going during her absence. There wasn't really much else that I could do. I couldn't ease her pain or share her struggle. In fact, aside from buying her a soft, fuzzy robe to wear at the hospital, it was the only concrete way that I could help my friend. But if I could keep up the routine, then all she'd have to do was rejoin me. That seemed a far easier task then letting it all slide and trying to pick up where we left off. So I continued to go it alone for the time she was out.

Amazingly, she wasn't out very long. In no time, it seemed as if she were back at it and we were partnering again, more energized than ever. Clearly, all the workouts we'd been doing leading up to her procedure had helped her rebound quickly and strongly.

Still, we hadn't left all of our old habits behind. If there was ever a time when one of us needed to miss a workout, because of an illness or vacation, the other would stay home as well and take advantage of the extra sleep time. Once, after skipping a day or so, Don called after us, incredulously, "You mean, just because one of you can't make it, the other one can't come either?"

When he put it that way, it did sound silly.

All of that changed when we began attending his kickboxing class on Wednesdays. We knew full well that if we ever missed a day—with good reason or not—we'd get a horrible ribbing. Granted, we didn't miss his class often, but just knowing we'd be harassed was enough incentive to get us into the gym solo on those rare occasions when the other one couldn't make it.

Then one Wednesday afternoon, I went shopping for a birthday card. As usual, my entire body was stiff and sore from that morning's class. As I lifted my arm to pull a card from the rack I felt a sharp, burning sensation deep within my shoulder. "Aaaah!" I moaned, grabbing my shoulder with my other hand. I literally could not raise my arm above my breastbone.

The following week, the pain was still present. I was faced with a dilemma: should I attend the class despite the injury or stay home? At that point, taking time off and falling behind Kris's progress was not something I wanted to do. Our friendly, competitive juices had started to flow.

I chose to go. Throughout the class, I modified the exercises so that I didn't use my right arm. I did one-arm jumping jacks, clutching my arm close to my side to keep it anchored. I marched in place when they dropped to the floor for push-ups. And I did punches with only my left arm. I made it through the class and it was still a good workout. For almost two months, I attended the class with my "broken wing" as Don called it. Eventually, I was able to use my right arm again and to slowly progress it in terms of strength and range of motion.

It was a valuable lesson for me. I learned that when you're injured, there are other exercises or activities that you can do. There are ways to modify your routine. Granted, it won't be the same. But rarely do you need to quit altogether. You may backslide some in terms of stamina, strength, or progress. However, when you are able to return full force, you'll quickly regain what was lost. And if it's your partner who's laid up, you can take the lead in maintaining the routine and staying on track, so she has something to return to, to look forward to, once her body mends. Speaking of staying on track, it's time for another ice bag and more Advil.

～ The Difference Between an Ouch, ～ an Injury, and an Interruption

An injury involves some part of your body being hurt to the degree that it can no longer perform the way it had been. Anytime you increase your intensity or try a new class or sport you will experience the ouch of sore muscles. One of the most important steps to take as you become more physically fit is to start to understand and recognize the differences between muscle soreness and the pain associated with an injury. It takes time to understand your own body—its limitations and tendencies— and to learn to spot the differences.

If you have not spent much time exercising, then the sensation of being sore—of being in pain—may be new to you. It usually lasts a few days, and is often worse on the second day after an activity. Don't shy away from activity because you feel sore. The best way to make the soreness go away is to continue to exercise or to walk. Extreme soreness can also be treated effectively by stretching (especially for the legs) or by an oral anti-inflammatory, such as ibuprofen.

Soreness is a normal reaction to the stress of exercise. It is usually felt on equal sides of the body. For example, if you start a running program it's likely both of your calves will be sore. The pain of an injury however will often continue throughout an activity, long after your muscles are warmed up. It can also seem more localized (on one calf rather than on both), though that's not always the case. Embrace sore muscles as a sign that you're progressing and working hard. Strive to understand when the sensation of pain is associated with an injury (rather than sore muscles) and needs to be treated or seen by a physician. It's always wise to seek the help of a doctor if you suspect a serious injury.

It is also important to learn how to describe your ouches and aches to your partner and others. This will help you conduct research on the Internet to gain insight into what's wrong as well as to accurately describe the symptoms and sensations to your doctor. Most times you will be able to locate an article or Internet site that perfectly matches your pain and outlines steps for you to follow in order to recover. So, take the time to listen to your body to try to determine whether it is an ouch or an injury. Again, when in doubt, consult a doctor.

If it's an injury, and depending upon the severity, you will need to allow that part of your body to rest in order to heal. For most basic muscle or tendon pulls and strains, a combination of rest, ice, and anti-inflammatory medication (such as Advil or Motrin) will do the trick. Resting the injury, however, does not necessarily mean that you need to quit your entire exercise routine. You may just need to modify your workouts in order to accommodate the injury. Sometimes doing the same exercises at a slower pace or intensity is all that's needed. The more you work out and are invested in your routine the more diligent you will be in researching your aches and pains because you will realize that when treated properly, most injuries do not need to impair your routine for long.

An interruption on the other hand is just that—it forces you to step away from your routine altogether for a period of time. It may be because of surgery or the birth of a baby. An interruption gives you no other choice but to take a hiatus from your routine. With an interruption, you need a plan. Talk with each other to decide and plot out how you can avoid having this temporary setback derail you permanently from your journey.

∽ Making a Comeback ∽

Treat each injury or interruption as an opportunity for you and your partner to evaluate and modify your program. It's the perfect time to make an assessment, revise the routine, and try something new. There are so many different classes and sports to try, that it's not too difficult to find ways to branch out. For example, if you are coming back from a leg injury, it may be the ideal chance to take a break from running and kickboxing, and head into the yoga and Pilates studio for the first time. Or, you may want to develop a revised routine that allows the injured partner to safely return to exercise but that also challenges the other partner. For example, a cycling class may allow one friend to do a non-weight-bearing exercise while the other can cycle as hard or as fast as she wants. Chances are that depending on the injury you will be able to come up with something that you both enjoy. Once you have a plan for your altered program, review it together and decide when you should kick it off.

As we found, if you face an injury or interruption that threatens to take one of you away from your routine for an extended period of time, it's critical for the "healthy" partner to continue on—for both your sakes. With a good partner at your side who can continue the routine, you'll find it is easier to jump back in close to where you left off, rather than both of you having to muster the motivation and discipline to start all over again. Plus, the healthy partner has ample reason to carry the torch solo.

During the comeback, be sure that the partner who's been sidelined does not return too quickly, however, and risk further injury or derailing the routine even longer. (This is an especially common problem with sports injuries, because often the pain disappears long before the muscle, tendon, or ligament is truly healed and operating at 100 percent. As a result, many people return to their workouts with full force, only to reinjure themselves.)

Like other challenges, injuries and interruptions will test the strength of your friendship, your commitment, and your resolve. If you can stay focused on maintaining the integrity of what you've built together, you will have earned the knowledge and the ability to weather any storm.

∽ **Notes** ∽

If you experience an injury, take some notes regarding what happened, what you felt, how it happened, and when it happened. Detail your days in recovery. Also make note of what you and your partner plan to do to stay on track and get you back on track once you've recovered. Mark your progress and make notes about what you'd do differently in the future. This information may prove helpful if you or your partner face a similar injury in the future.

CHAPTER 7

TAKING IT TO
THE NEXT LEVEL

ERHAPS NO OTHER change will foster dramatic improvements in your fitness level—and move you through the body
and mind phases of your wellness journey—than increasing
the intensity of your workouts. This may translate into walking faster, or
trying a new activity such as running or cycling, or pushing yourself to
do a few more push-ups. Increasing the intensity simply means working
much harder than you've been working before. You can increase the intensity of any activity. It is by constantly challenging yourself that you'll
see tremendous gains in physical strength and endurance, as well as in
self-confidence, mental focus, and resolve. Each time you increase your
intensity—and meet that challenge head-on—your body, mind, and
soul adapt to the added stress so that in short order they will be ready for
more challenges. It's an amazing phenomenon.

∼ Kris Looks Back ∼

In our early months at the gym, we could easily talk the other into *de-
creasing* the intensity of our workouts. "I didn't sleep well last night." Or,
"I started my period." Or, "I'm getting ready to start my period." Or, "I
just finished my period." It didn't take much prompting for the other
partner to chime in, "That's fine with me. I feel like a gentle cycle ride

too." So we would talk and pedal casually for thirty minutes before heading home.

That began to change after we started going to Don's kickboxing class every Wednesday morning. By Thursday we would have to roll ourselves off the bed, because sitting up was so painful. Eventually, after several months, our bodies started to adjust and to respond. Our shapes changed. I'd often do a double take when I passed the mirror. It didn't look like "me." My arms and back became more defined. My silhouette became slimmer. Clothing started to fit differently. But more important, my mind and soul began to crave the challenge and intensity of the workout. The more determined we became, the more Don was cheering us on, encouraging us, pushing us to work hard, and then even harder.

Four years later, so much has changed. For many years, my husband always encouraged me to work out. But I had no interest or I had lost my way on how to begin. Today, he thinks I am nuts. "All that running isn't good for you," he'll say. Or, "It's okay to sleep in one day past 5 a.m." But workouts are a priority. I crave exercise.

Now we arrive as soon as the gym opens. We grab every minute of available time to exercise and only head home in order to get our children off to school—often racing there so we won't be late. If one of us can stay longer than the other, it's cause for serious envy.

As our intensity increased, so too, did our individual determination and dedication. In the early days, if one of us took a vacation, it would derail the routine for both of us. Not anymore. Now, whoever goes on vacation tries to work out as much as possible because she knows the partner is maintaining her routine at home. Exercise lies at the heart of who we are now—regardless of where we are. Truth is, I'm just not the same me when I don't work out.

∼ Kim Looks Back ∼

One day, after a couple of years in Don's class, I came home brimming with glee. "I can jump rope for twenty minutes straight!" I reported to my husband.

He responded, eyebrows raised, "The next thing you're going to tell me is that you want to train for the Iditarod." (The Iditarod Trail Sled

Dog Race is a grueling event that covers the frozen wilderness of Alaska and spans many days, if not weeks.) It was funny, but he had a point. There was no telling what we were going to come home to announce next. Because with each physical challenge we tackled, each milestone we reached, we kept wanting more, more, more.

Once we began to experience and understand the cycle of intensity— the links between mind, body, and soul—something sparked. We were driven to find new challenges. Our fitness pursuits catapulted to a whole different level. We respected challenges. Fear no longer stood in our way. And failure no longer loomed as an issue. Instead, we simply needed a different plan. We needed to find a way to succeed. The doors began to fly wide open. We could run a marathon. We could write a book. We could change careers. We could become personal trainers. We could open a business. We could help make a difference in the lives of others. Anything, everything seemed possible.

Initially, after increasing the intensity of our workouts through Don's kickboxing class, the most noticeable changes were in our bodies—from our figures to how efficiently we burned calories to how much we would sweat during a workout. But the greatest transformation that resulted from our time with Don involved the mental resolve we gained. When you push yourself, time after time, beyond your comfort level, beyond your current abilities, and you start to see results, you begin to understand the process of self-improvement. *There is no substitute for putting the time in and doing the work.* It's that work that leads to results. So, when you finish a class—despite the many moments you wanted to quit—your pride and perspective change. When you accomplish that time after time, your mind is transformed. You start to realize that you *can* do something hard, something physically demanding, and focus in such a way that you push yourself through until you get to the other side. That process is what makes you mentally tough.

When you are mentally tough, you will not be afraid to tackle a myriad of challenges. That toughness will spill into other areas of your life. It will help you stand firm and tall. It will make you want to treat yourself better and to demand better treatment from others. It will enable you to put the small, daily annoyances into their proper perspective. It will give you clarity, so that you can move purposefully through your days. You will begin to act, rather than react to life.

∿ Find Someone to Lead You ∿ to Intensity

For some reason, it is difficult to push ourselves. Perhaps it's human nature. Most people tend to stop themselves just shy of the hardest challenge. We're no different. Over the years, it's true that we had to do the actual work and put in the effort. We had to manage and maintain our routine. We had to keep showing up. But we credit Don with inspiring us and allowing us to arrive at fitness levels we never even dreamed we'd reach. Without him, you would not be reading this book.

So, while the friendship can help lead you to consistency, you may need to find someone who can truly motivate you to push yourselves beyond your limits. Because personal trainers can be expensive to hire on an ongoing basis (two to three times a week), some of the best people to turn to are class instructors. A good instructor can motivate you to do more. So if you and your friend think you will struggle to push yourselves to new heights, consider taking a class.

Be diligent in finding the right instructor and the class that works for you. In the end, the right instructor is worth her weight in gold. Find the instructor who can spur you beyond what you think you're capable of. That will mean the difference between whether or not you start to realize all of the benefits and gifts that can be gained through your hard work.

∿ Motivation—What's Your ∿ Golden Carrot?

Motivation is critical at all phases in your fitness journey. It can become even more crucial when you face challenging workouts in your effort to increase the intensity. Pushing yourself will test your fortitude. To succeed, you need to understand the role that motivation plays in your routine. Motivation is an individual trait. Some people have been blessed with a strong, inner discipline and desire. Unfortunately, we're not those people. And you probably aren't either.

However, being born without an innate need to exercise doesn't mean you can't manufacture motivation. After all, that's the entire crux of this book: doing it together so you stay motivated to continue doing it together.

In analyzing what gets us going and keeps us going, we've come to the conclusion that we draw our motivation and inspiration from three principles. These elements, or some combination of them, are always present, underlying our routine and spawning our motivation

- **We need each other.** We've stressed this from the beginning. We've been able to achieve a high degree of physical fitness largely because when we socialize we are nurturing aspects of our mental health. We may not spend our entire workout chatting, but more often than not we get some opportunity to connect—to get our fix of one another. Many times we use our warm-up and cooldown time to chat, and then turn our focus to getting "in the zone." Feeling strong mentally helps to motivate you to be more physical, and vice versa. Mind and body are intrinsically linked and can do wonders for one another, when both receive the attention they deserve. As friends, we also need each other to motivate us to continue getting better. When one works hard, the other will respond by working just as hard. When one wants to try something new, the other will follow suit. Neither one of us wants to be left behind, so we always strive to keep up with each other. We bring out the best in each other.
- **We need an instructor who works us hard.** Many workout fiends don't need an instructor to push them through another set of push-ups. But we do. We love having a class with an instructor who will make us "leave it on the floor" as they say. Again, the importance of having the right instructor, one who motivates, inspires, and encourages you in just the right ways cannot be emphasized enough. If you don't leave the room wanting more and waiting to return (regardless of how tired or sore you may be), then that particular instructor isn't the one for you. Seek out the ones who get you jazzed about the workout.
- **We need a goal.** We have learned over time that we are both indisputably goal-oriented. When we're focused on a goal, we're very intense. Once we set a goal we don't waiver, and we have an amazing amount of discipline. Through the pursuit of goals we have been able to reach higher fitness levels. Without goals, we can feel somewhat slack, unfocused, and far less intense—even

though we're still getting up every morning, doing more and working harder than ever before. However, it wasn't until we were well on our way to being fit, that we realized this need. So in the beginning, don't concern yourself too much with goals. As you see progress and your perspective shifts, as you build your own time line of milestones, you too may naturally start to crave setting fitness goals to keep you going.

Perhaps it's the mix of these three elements that work best. After all, it's hard to constantly have fitness goals—particularly if you're training for something, such as a race. It's unreasonable to expect to maintain an intense training schedule for an endless period of time. On the other hand, constantly having social time during your workouts impairs your ability to rev up the intensity. You simply can't chat while you're working your hardest. If you can, then you're not working hard enough. Last, it would be impossible to find just the right classes with the ideal instructors at the exact times you need to exercise. So you can see how having a mix of these elements, addressed at any given time, can work well to inspire your fitness efforts.

The final aspect of motivation that must be understood is its ability to ebb and flow. Even when you are intently focused on training to reach a specific goal—such as getting ready for an event or a race—your daily motivation will rise and fall. Some days you will feel invincible, able to work as hard as a champion. Other days, the last thing you will want to do is lace up your shoes. Whether you're training for something big or just trying to keep to a routine, you need to recognize that your motivation to do so will come and go. You need to find ways to bridge the gaps. That's why we stress the importance of being in this adventure with your friend. Simply having to meet her somewhere will be what gets you out the door. The partnership forms the foundation for all of your pursuits. The various motivating forces form the structure and the frame for what you're building together. Having an instructor can be like having a foreman around to encourage you to work harder—when all you want to do is sit down and have a cup of coffee.

Finally, always remember that even a bad workout day will leave you feeling better, physically and mentally, than a day without a workout.

When one or all of these elements come together to compensate for lagging motivation, it keeps you going. Recognize what is at work and when, and realize that you must find a way to continue your routine despite your waning desire.

∽ How to Take It to the Next Level ∽

Here are some ways you can increase the intensity of your workouts so that you're enhancing your cardiovascular capacity and stamina:

- **Increase the pace of your activity.** You can pick up the pace by simply walking faster or by adding some gentle jogging. Try a few different approaches. You can increase your overall pace slightly to moderately. Or, you can increase your pace dramatically for a short time or distance (such as a half-minute, full-minute, or two-minute period) followed by a period (such as a minute) when you return to a more comfortable pace, letting your heart rate and breathing recover.
- **Increase the number of times each week that you work out (frequency).** Another way to take it to the next level is to work out more often. This may require you and your friend to reassess your schedules and to see where you can grab more snatches of time together. As always, try to take this step together if at all possible, so that you continue to share the experience.
- **Increase the length of time that you work out (duration).** Even adding ten or fifteen minutes more to your workouts can do wonders for helping you rev things up. That's enough time to add a new activity or a few new exercises, or to simply do something you enjoy a bit longer.
- **Take an aerobics or cycling class.** Adding just one class per week to your routine can help. Classes also offer a more structured approach, which ensures a proper warm-up and cooldown.
- **Pick a machine with programmed workouts.** Most machines have programmed workouts, which allow you to choose options such as intervals or hills. Experiment with the different machines and workout options to find one that you like.

- **Sign up for an event and put a training plan together.** There are a host of running, cycling, and multisport races for a variety of different fitness levels. Choose an entry-level point for any event—meaning, start with a 5K rather than a marathon. Then conduct research or find a credentialed coach to help you put a buddy training program together. Then be sure to give yourselves ample time to train.

As you increase the intensity of your workouts, you may find that what's hard for you will not necessarily be hard for your friend. That's because your bodies are different. You have different shapes and may be different sizes. Your body will have its own core strengths and weaknesses. Don't worry about who is better at any given exercise. Instead, use it as an opportunity to help nudge each other along the path of improvement. One may be naturally stronger at push-ups. That's great, because the other person will work harder in order to keep up and arrive at the same level. The other person might be a stronger cycler. If so, she will take the lead in setting the tone for pace and cadence. You will find that you alternate between taking the lead in those activities for which you are best suited and being led. Regardless of which activities feel more natural to you given your physique, consistency pays off. With consistency, intensity, and proper form, anyone and everyone can improve their abilities.

∿ **Feeling Winded** ∿

As you push yourself to new levels, you will huff and puff your way there. That painful, gripping sensation deep in your chest is the first big step to getting your heart and your lungs stronger. While it's a good sign that you're working hard, you need to be sure—as with everything— that you take it slow. Learn to listen to your body and all the signals it sends. Learn to trust your instincts. It's okay to push your lungs' capacity beyond their current rate for short periods of time. But you want to be sure to give your lungs a chance to recover, so you can get your breathing back under control.

If you feel too winded in an aerobics class, simply modify the movement. You can march in place until you catch your breath. Or, do the leg movement without the arms. If you're in a cycling class, slow your spinning pace down a bit or lighten the resistance on the bike. Whatever you do, don't merely stop to try to catch your breath. Keep doing some type of movement at a moderate pace, so that you continue to progress. Strive to keep your breathing controlled and relaxed. Practice purposeful breathing. If you are consistent, you will see improvements quickly. In time you'll even be able to try new activities far more easily than before.

∾ Sore Muscles ∾

As we've mentioned in earlier chapters, whenever you try a new activity or increase the intensity of your workouts, you'll experience sore muscles. Depending on how challenging the activity was, your muscles may be so sore that you feel as if you can't walk or it hurts so much to lift your arms that you can't shampoo your hair. As painful as they can be at times, sore muscles can be a good thing—a sign that you're pushing yourself and working harder.

∾ One Activity Does Not Necessarily ∾ Prepare You for Another

If you do one activity for a prolonged period of time, your body adjusts to it and will no longer experience soreness (unless you increase the intensity of that activity). But as soon as you try a new activity, you'll be sore and tired all over again. So if you've been doing aerobics for months and you decide to start running, you'll feel a host of new aches, pains, and sore muscles. That's because fitness in one area does not necessarily translate to another—although it's still easier than starting from scratch. Best of all, if you reach the point where you are eager to seek out new activities and to take on new physical challenges, then there's no doubt you are well on your way to achieving peak fitness—mind, body, and soul.

∽ **Notes** ∽

Keep a list of instructors and classes that are recommended to you by friends or people at the gym. When you're ready to alter your routine, consider taking one of these classes.

List three fitness goals that have crossed your mind (e.g., run a 5K race, become a yoga instructor). When you're ready to increase your intensity (at any point in your journey) look to this list as a great place to begin. Chat with your partner about shared goals, first steps, and plans.

CHAPTER 8

STARTING TO FEEL FIT

EELING FIT is a relative term. Much will depend upon how "unfit" you feel at the start of your journey. Starting to experience improvements in your fitness level can begin almost immediately as you track your daily and weekly gains in endurance, distance, time, or quality of your workouts. Or, perhaps you're feeling a greater sense of calm and are falling asleep faster and sleeping more soundly. This chapter will focus on the various stages of becoming fit—all those little signs coming from within your soul, your body, and your mind, that tell you that you're on the right path.

∼ Kris Looks Back ∼

Kim had just left me to go to her starting corral, and I was thinking how inexperienced we were regarding races. We had no idea that based on our estimated finish times we would have to start our first half-marathon race without each other. But so it was that I was standing all alone in my corral nervously waiting for the race to begin. As I was stretching, I was checking out the racers all around me. Looking around, my confidence began to grow. I look as fit as these runners, I thought. Could it be that I look like a runner? It was that day, as we ran the half-marathon race, that I gained another piece of the fitness puzzle: the body piece. My body had morphed into an athlete's body—or at least closer to one than it had ever been in the past.

Yet when I look back on our journey I realized that the first piece of the fitness puzzle to fall into place—the soul piece—happened during our "walking-talking program." During those walking days we had found the time to reflect on our current life and dare to dream about other wants we possessed that were going unfulfilled. I discovered that I no longer loved my career. I wanted a flexible schedule to pursue other interests, interests that I knew I must have deep inside, but had not had time to dare think about. Eventually, I left an unsatisfying career of ten plus years to try something new from home.

During our walking phase, I also slowly began to get in touch with my body. I learned to know it better. In doing so, I discovered that my health was still not perfect. Prompted by a poor recovery from my first surgery, I knew that I wanted and needed to be more aggressive in taking care of myself. That's when I ventured into the gym with the hopes of getting my body stronger.

The final piece of the fitness puzzle—the mind piece—fell into place only after my soul was fulfilled and my body was healthy and strong. Once my soul and body were in sync, all my decisions became more mindful and easier. I wanted to eat correctly to improve how my body performed. I no longer wanted to skip workouts or to work out only in an effort to lose weight. And I learned to accept such limitations as not being able to have another child and to refocus my energy on those things that I could change and improve.

∿ Kim Looks Back ∿

By late 2001, we had spent several months in Don's kickboxing class. While the numbers on my scale hadn't changed much, people were starting to react and comment on my figure when they saw me. Most assumed that I was losing weight, but the truth is, my shape was changing rather than there being any change in my weight.

I noticed it too. When I passed a mirror, I had to do a double take because I didn't really recognize my shape any more. I seemed far more narrow than I had been and a lot less "hippy." It took some getting used to.

I then noticed changes in my upper body. I could feel my muscles taking shape and noticed small bulges near my biceps. It was such a concrete change, that I would often mindlessly rub the side of my arm just to feel the indentation near my triceps. I had never at any point in my life ever had muscles in my arms (or anywhere for that matter).

Over more time, I realized that we could last longer and longer in Don's classes. Because his class was so hard, each week meant meeting the challenge head-on, rising to the occasion, and not giving up. Aside from giving birth, I had never been challenged in this way physically before. Eventually we were able to do his entire class without stopping. Even when Don kept ramping it up, we were able to hang. My body was performing at levels I never imagined possible for me. I could feel my confidence soar. I began to shed the image of myself as the little girl who was always picked last for a team. I began to understand that there was a distinct difference between having athletic ability and being fit. Even if I wasn't born athletic, I could still become incredibly fit.

As my body continued to change, becoming more muscular and toned, it seemed as if people I met viewed me as athletic or (even funnier) as a "naturally" thin person. They'd comment, "Someone like you doesn't need to worry about weight." Little did they know how funny that comment sounds to me.

That's when it sunk in that there was a big difference between being "thin" and being "fit." When I sought thinness, by way of diets only, at any given moment I was perched on the possibility of failing. Only if I maintained the weight loss did I feel successful. Thus, that feeling of accomplishment could be dashed instantly after a single weekend of parties or eating out. Even gaining a pound would have me feeling bad about myself. Let alone experiencing a five-pound (or more) swing.

Becoming fit started to change that too. It gave me so many reasons to be proud, so many accomplishments to hang my hat on that a five-pound weight gain after a week's vacation became a mere annoyance rather than an entire blow to my self-esteem. I still hate to put on excess pounds and have my clothes fit snugly. But being fit means that as soon as I return home from vacation, I simply get back into my routine by going for a ten-mile run! Nothing can diminish my ability to do that. With better fitness I began to have more to feel proud of, more accomplishments to help me keep things in perspective, and more reasons to step away from the scale and stop living life by the numbers.

All of these milestones along our journey led to my growing ability to handle the smaller things in life with greater ease. As I started to feel more confident, I felt less anxiety. I began to believe in my own wants, needs, likes, and dislikes. I looked less and less to others for validation of what I wanted out of life. I cared a bit less about what others thought. I began to make conscious decisions about how I wanted to spend my time and with whom. I was able to see what I wanted versus what I had often done only to please others. My own values and sense of beliefs began to crystallize. A sense of calm enveloped my days. I seemed to move through them with more clarity and purpose.

The workouts gave me an ideal physical outlet from which to grow and change. The daily opportunities for Kris and I to connect and chat, gave me an outlet that allowed my mind and my soul to grow, to change, to flourish.

Because the changes were so subtle and occurred over time, I often only noticed them with hindsight. I'd think, "Wow, I would have freaked out over that a while back." Or, "Hey, that problem didn't keep me up all night tossing and turning with worry." As more times like that happened I began to pay careful attention to how different my days seemed now. Life had a more natural, easy rhythm to it. Everything—body, mind, soul—seemed to fit together nicely.

∽ What Does It Feel Like to Feel Fit? ∽

There is no greater feeling than to set a goal and accomplish it. Even better is to set a goal that seems outrageous, to set out on a plan and then do it. When you feel fit in mind, body, and soul and you are able to share that feeling and experience with a friend, you develop a belief that you can accomplish anything. There is tremendous freedom gained through confidence and companionship. You may gain freedom from the realization that being fit and being thin are not the same. You may gain freedom from realizing that you can set boundaries and choose to say no without feeling guilty or feeling like a failure. You may gain freedom to explore new dreams and to let go of old obstacles blocking your way. When you are set free, no longer do you need to listen to or be influenced by the naysayers (of which there are many!) Instead, you move forward pursuing *your* passions, *your* vision of your life, with a drive and determination that you never realized you possessed.

∼ Some of the Signs You May Notice ∼

You may notice a host of signs as you become fitter. These are just some signs we noticed in our own lives.

- **You'll see concrete, albeit subtle, improvements.** The first sign you will notice with each passing week is that you no longer become winded walking up stairs or up a hill. Your muscles will stop being sore. You may notice that you sleep better on the nights you walk or exercise. Perhaps lifting groceries or a toddler gets a bit easier. Or, you can stand for longer periods of time without your legs getting tired.

  Some of the initial fitness gains are also not necessarily related to physical accomplishments. Getting into a routine for an extended period of time is a tremendous accomplishment. These types of milestones can quickly add up to great rewards. It's a good idea to take note of these improvements and changes in your life, in order to remind yourselves of how far you've come. It's a great boost when you're feeling frustrated or down about your progress, to step back and see the big picture—to see where you are versus where you once were. Eventually, believe it or not, you won't be able to remember a time when you were inactive and you will wonder why it was so difficult to start to exercise in the first place.

- **You'll notice the reactions of others.** Another sign that you're on the right track is that friends and family will make comments. They may notice some weight loss or that your body is changing. Unfortunately, not all of their comments will be kind. In fact, they may be rather unsupportive. Thus, you may have to ignore a snide remark or two. Realize that as you improve yourself, others may feel jealous or begrudge you those changes. Worse, some of the people you care about most might surprise you with their reaction. Work to stay focused on what you really want and to ignore people who aren't supportive of what you do.

Often their comments will be subtle, such as, "I wouldn't get up so early to work out if it meant going to bed early and taking time away from my husband." When people make these types of comments, they are designed to make themselves feel better (and justify their lack of commitment) and to make you feel guilty for yours.

Any time you find you're excited about your routine, or your accomplishments, you may also find that you're a target for unsolicited reproach. Ignore the types of comments that are designed to make you reconsider what you're doing. Have faith that you're on course; don't let others steer you wrong.

- **You'll need a daily change of clothing.** Another sign that your fitness level is improving and that you're really working hard is that you can barely stand how drenched you are and how bad you smell when you're done. It's as if you can't get your clothes off and into the washer fast enough. If you started your walking journey wearing big cotton T-shirts over tights or shorts, in time you may realize that you're in need of a new outfit because those big Ts get saturated in stinky sweat and hang down to your knees. As your exercise routine evolves so too will your workout clothing. Each change—whether you switch from T-shirts to tank tops or from wearing cotton to wicking fabrics—will mark a new level in your fitness quest.

- **You'll primp and preen.** Let's face it, as you start to notice dramatic changes in your body it's hard to ignore them. This is especially true if you've struggled with your weight. When you start to change your body, it's as if you need constant reassurance that "*Yes*, this is still me!" You may catch yourself in the bathroom, buck naked, flexing your biceps and triceps as if you were Ms. Universe. You may be amazed (and proud!) of what you see. You may also start to choose clothing—like tank tops—that show off the results of all your hard work. Don't be shy! You deserve to be confident and proud of how far you've come. Again, enjoy and appreciate the compliments that come your way, and ignore the whispers behind your back.

- **You'll notice it seems to get worse, before it gets better.** While it's exciting to see results, sometimes when your body goes through major changes, it can look kind of funky! And it will seem to get worse before it gets better. That's because losing (or gaining) inches in one area may make another area look horrendous. Or, you might lose inches in one wacky place and not in another. As your legs tighten up your bottom may appear flabby. When your bottom firms up it may seem wider and, oddly enough, higher than it was. If your waist trims a bit, you'll realize that you actually do have large hips. Do not become discouraged as you see all these changes. Try to avoid becoming highly critical of body parts that do not yet appear toned. Although it is healthy to assess your figure and to design your workouts to complement your desired results, it is also important to remember the progress you have already made. One way to maintain your perspective is to document progress by taking measurements of your legs, bottom, hips, abs, chest, and arms. Take measurements roughly twice a year, to give yourself enough time to make lasting changes. Another option is to have someone take photos of you. Photos are a great way to really "see" progress, since often it's only in photos that we recognize how different we may look.

Your body may also cycle through a series of radical changes followed by a plateau. You'll notice major changes almost overnight and then, just as suddenly, your body will quit changing and stay the same for a while. Changing your routine and taking it to the next level can shock your body into its next round of changes.

- **You'll look for other challenges.** As your fitness level increases, you will start to contemplate how you can challenge yourself more. Perhaps you'll ponder entering a race or event. Or, you'll have the confidence to try different and perhaps unconventional activities such as rock climbing or kayaking. By all means, take on the challenge, but do it wisely. Conduct research to find a solid training program. Contact an instructor or trainer to introduce you to the activity safely. Your ultimate goal as you take on new challenges should be to stay injury free and to have a positive experience—so that you can continue to try new things. Above everything, however, is to remember to seek activities that you and your friend can do together. After all, that's how you got

this far in the first place—it will be more rewarding and memorable to have your friend beside you every step of the way.
- You'll become "obsessed."

> *Obsessed is just a word the lazy use to describe the dedicated.*
> —ANONYMOUS

At some point, although we're not sure when, we became highly dedicated to our fitness pursuits—so much so, that we even call ourselves obsessed. Today, we're fairly certain that we'd be able to keep up our routine without each other, though we wouldn't want to try. Now, missing a day, let alone several days, is cause for dismay. It has become a higher priority than most other things in our lives, and we move heaven and earth to squeeze it in, still sticking to the early morning hours because there are fewer chances we'll get derailed. When blowing off a workout no longer feels good or when you find ways to work out while on vacation, then you're dedicated to fitness. When you scrutinize the athletes you come across in life, and ask yourself "I wonder how heavy a weight she's lifting to get those biceps?" then you're probably obsessed. When you pore over magazines like *Runner's World*, *Outside*, and *Her Sports*, soaking up all the latest and greatest fitness info you can find, you're hooked. Welcome to the club!
- **You'll begin to apply the discipline skills you've cultivated to other areas of your life.** After you realize that you have, in fact, become a highly disciplined person you'll begin to transfer those skills into the rest of your days and the decisions you make—whether that means eating healthier or standing firm and demanding better treatment from others.
- **Then, "fit" simply becomes who you are.** Once you've achieved these milestones, being fit becomes who you are. It will be how you think of yourself—so much so that you can't imagine *not* staying fit. In time, you will notice that people you meet will think of you as being strong, being fit. You'll be able to tell by the things they say, the comments they make. They won't know the "old" you. Gone will be the days when you struggled to be consistent. Gone will be the days when you could easily be derailed from working out, or when you could let months or years go by

without walking into the gym. Even if you get derailed by illness or by life's interruptions, your first thoughts will be figuring out how and when you can get back to your routine. You'll no longer fear the soreness or the challenge of getting back to where you once were, you'll just know it's part of the process.

If you want to become the fit woman described in this chapter, then dog-ear this page, return to it again and again as you continue on your journey, until it describes the very essence of who you are. And if this page is worn with wear, has been dog-eared a hundred times, and you've become the woman described in these pages, then congratulations! We're thrilled you've succeeded in your quest. You have much to be proud of, but then you already know that, don't you?

∼ Notes ∼

Use this space to celebrate all of your fitness gains throughout your journey. Start tracking from the beginning with all the small improvements you notice. Or, if you've been working hard for a while, think back and write down some notes to help you chronicle your milestones. You will be amazed each time you review the list to see how far you've come.

_____

_____

_____

_____

_____

_____

_____

_____

_____

_____

CHAPTER 9

CHANGING YOUR
EATING HABITS

P ART OF BECOMING FIT certainly involves eating healthier
and making wiser food choices. But developing and applying the discipline and the skills necessary to accomplish this
on a daily basis, will come during the final phases of your fitness journey.
This chapter explores that process.

There seem to be two types of people in the world. Those who eat to
live. And those who live to eat. Those who eat to live usually only eat
when they're hungry and rarely overeat to the point where they'd be uncomfortable or "feel stuffed." They don't struggle with their weight.
Those who live to eat however, struggle daily. They struggle at every
meal. They struggle to control their eating, or to avoid snacks, or to eliminate carbs, or to count calories. They struggle with their weight. They
struggle to know whether or not they are even hungry. They struggle to
avoid eating for emotional reasons, such as stress, sadness, boredom, and
even happiness. Sound familiar?

If it does, you're not alone. More and more people fit into this category
than ever before. Why? Because whether it's the availability of super-size
fries or the message to "finish everything on your plate," our society has
succeeded in reprogramming us. We are bombarded with messages about
food and eating—from constant advertising to fast-food joints on every
corner to 7-Elevens that serve anything from hard-boiled eggs to chili

dogs. Moreover, it's quick and easy to satisfy the cravings we all have. Plus, we turn to food for a host of reasons, although few if any have anything to do with the primary reason we need to eat: to fuel our bodies. As we've conditioned ourselves to eat at times other than when we're hungry, we've actually lost our ability to identify the hunger sensation. With the notion of food front and center in our lives each and every day, it's incredibly hard to eat *only* when you're hungry.

With all the diets on the market and perhaps with all the diets you may have tried yourself (assuming of course, that you struggle with your weight), then you already know *what* you need to do to lose pounds. The fact is weight control is all about calories in and calories out. Again, you already know that. You've read enough books about what you need to do. Perhaps you've even invested in structured weight-loss programs. If you're like most dieters, you've probably even succeeded to some extent, if only for a short time.

What's usually missing for most people is the understanding of how to succeed long term, how to succeed at making lifelong changes. Why is it so hard to succeed for the long haul? Because, diets by their very nature leave us feeling deprived. There's really nothing empowering about being on a diet. It's a black-and-white, win-or-lose proposition. As long as you're "losing" weight you'll feel like a winner. Only as long as you're depriving yourself (because that's what it feels like to give up the foods and the portions you love) will you feel successful. But any slight change—whether it's a natural fluctuation in weight or a "slip" at dinner or a week's vacation—can quickly make you feel like a failure. Your entire self-esteem is tightly wrapped around every little decision, every morsel, every meal. And so, for the entire time that you place yourself on a diet, you teeter on the fence between success and failure. Worse, when you feel you've failed, it's easy to soothe your emotions by turning to food. Of course, that only perpetuates the cycle.

Is it possible to get off the diet cycle and get back to how nature intended you to be—so that you eat primarily when you're hungry? Can you reprogram yourself to get back in touch with knowing *what* your body needs, *when* it needs it? Is it possible to become someone who eats healthily but who doesn't constantly feel deprived?

We believe it is.

∼ Kim Looks Back ∼

I first started to turn to food to soothe my emotions when I was in fifth grade. In the middle of that year I switched schools and started attending the local public school a few blocks from my house. Each day, I walked home and had roughly two hours of time to kill before my mom got home from work. I would plop myself down in front of the TV and serve up a heaping bowl of vanilla ice cream. Sometimes I sprinkled Nestle's Quick on it. Sometimes I drizzled chocolate syrup over it. And sometimes I ate it plain. After I was done, I usually went to the freezer again and served up another bowl full. I was eating mostly because I was bored and also a bit lonely. Eating gave me something to do. And it was a great complement to watching *I Love Lucy* reruns.

Because I never participated in any organized sports, as I got older I began to move farther and farther away from exercise as I outgrew my childhood loves like biking, foursquare, and roller-skating. Heading into middle school and early high school, the only exercise I got was walking to and from friends' houses. As a result, once I turned sixteen and started driving, I managed to completely eliminate all exercise and activity from my life. (Which seemed fine at the time, because frankly, I hated to exercise.)

In addition to eating when I was home alone and bored, I added social eating to my list of pursuits. During my junior and senior years in high school, friends and I went to McDonald's nearly every single day. I always ordered a Big Mac, french fries, and a chocolate shake. If we didn't head to McDonald's we went for Chinese food. Or, if we were somehow stranded at the school cafeteria, we'd order chocolate shakes for lunch. Quickly, the pounds piled on. As they did, I grappled with trying to lose them. That marked my entry into the world of weight-loss products and solutions, as I tried everything from Dexatrim and Slim-Fast to Weight Watchers and NutriSystem, and far more extreme approaches like binging, purging, and starvation.

The trouble was nothing worked long term. As soon as I had a measure of success, something lured me back to old habits and patterns. Worse was the fact that I kept picking up more bad habits to go along with the ones I'd already established. By the time I hit college, my roommates and I were frequenting all-you-can-eat restaurants and stopping at the twenty-four-hour Hardees at 3:00 a.m. for a hot ham 'n cheese before we went to bed. When I'd hit a threshold of tolerance for the bigger me I'd become, I'd react feverishly using a frantic approach with the hopes I'd see some drastic results.

I see now all those attempts to become thin were doomed from the start. Knowing what I do today, it seems as if I always had the cart before the horse. I was desperate to get the weight-loss wagon moving, without having a way to lead it. It was only after becoming more physically active and consistent in my exercise, that my whole relationship with food was altered, albeit slowly. Fitness led the way.

Of course, not at first. Initially, when we started our walking program, I gave myself full justification to eat whatever I wanted, whenever I wanted. I would think "I deserved to eat that! After all, I worked out!" Food was my reward.

Several months after we started running, that approach flip-flopped. I would catch myself having more self-control when it came to food and thinking, "I'm not going to eat that. I worked out too hard to blow it all on that." And yet, on the occasions when I wanted to treat myself to something or to simply lower my guard, I could also easily say, "I deserve that, after all, I'm still working out." It was a nice balance. Best of all, I didn't feel like an utter failure each time I ate something "I shouldn't." That's because I finally had exercise fueling my self-esteem and sense of accomplishment. I had the confidence of knowing that the exercise was always burning calories. No longer did everything (how I felt about and viewed myself) hinge on what I ate or what I weighed. Even gaining a few pounds wasn't the end of the world. It didn't signal a huge backslide, where five pounds led to twenty. Instead, I knew that my workout routine would provide the extra discipline and incentive I needed to get me back on track. That eliminated that dooming sense of failure and feeling out of control. It was both freeing and empowering. Plus, since the exercise helped me cope with stress and everyday life in general, I naturally turned less and less to food for comfort.

As we progressed along the fitness track, performance and endurance became larger goals for us. That prompted us to learn more about the relationship between food and how it makes your body feel. As much as I knew about dieting, all the dos and donts, there was an entire facet of nutrition-based performance that I knew nothing about (much of which conflicts with what popular diets espouse). It was a whole different way of looking at food, as well as looking at the mind and body connection.

∾ Kris Looks Back ∾

At a holiday cocktail party in late 2002, I was having a conversation with a former collegiate rower and her husband (who had once been her coach). They were laughing about how strict he had been regarding the rowing team's eating and drinking choices. No fast food, no sodas, no alcohol. Having never asked my body to perform at that level, I was curious if all the food and drink choices really made a difference. Without hesitation she stated, "Absolutely!" Kim and I had just decided that we would start training for a half-marathon race. I was very nervous about my ability to complete this race. The longest I had ever run was a 10K (or 6.2 miles).

The conversation that night stuck with me. It made me start to question and consider my eating habits. Could the right foods really make a big difference in how my body performed? Could foods really affect how I felt? I was willing to give it a try.

At that point, my body mass index (or BMI) was in the appropriate range for my height and age with regard to my weight, although it was on the higher end of the range. Honestly, I would have liked to have lost some weight, but I just could not seem to make it happen. But armed with the stretch goal of doing the half marathon, I decided to tune up my eating habits.

The main changes I made were to drink more water, eat more fiber, have smaller portion sizes, eat healthier snacks, and cut out any snacking after dinner. I did lose weight. But what was more amazing was that when I followed my new habits, I felt awesome during my workouts. Not only did I feel stronger, but I had more energy and endurance. And whenever I slipped, my workouts seemed much more difficult and I felt sluggish.

Feeling the difference in how your body performs when it's fueled correctly is a powerful tool to use for weight maintenance. Today, my weight will increase and decrease depending on the type of event or goal I am training for, but in general, I eat healthier because I prefer how it makes my body feel.

∽ Put the Horse before the Cart ∽

If you have been overeating and living to eat, then changing your behavior will be difficult. How difficult will depend upon where you are in your fitness quest. Again, take a moment to look back on our time line. You'll see that taking control of our eating, being mindful of what we ate, did not come for us until late in our journey. At the time it was the next logical step. By then, we had the tools and discipline to carry it through.

If you've progressed along the fitness continuum from *nurturing your soul* to *challenging your body* to *cultivating the power of your mind*, then you might be ready for change. If you've achieved that much, then you have already acquired what it takes to make long-lasting changes in terms of how you approach food. As we said, you already have the knowledge. Through fitness you've gained the discipline and resolve. So, set a course and get started!

If you're not that far along in your fitness journey, then the challenge of changing your eating may best be saved for later, when you've developed the tools and skills you'll need to succeed. That's because if it's early in your journey, you likely have a host of reasons to explain why you are where you are today: "I had three children in four years," "I had two C-sections," "I have a career that requires me to eat out all the time," "I've always been heavy." In addition to the excuses, your body is actually craving the foods that it's used to getting. So, changing your eating habits will seem impossible until you *change your reasons for wanting to have healthier habits.* "To lose weight" or "to look better" is simply not enough of a substantive reason or an incentive to sustain long-term change. That point is so important, we need to say it again: "To lose weight" or "to look better" is simply not enough of a substantive reason or an incentive to sustain long-term change. You need to seduce your body and your mind into change. The way you do that is to get your body moving.

It seems so simple: to get your body moving.

Granted, we fully understand that taking those first few steps toward establishing a routine is a huge battle. After all, this entire book centers around how you can seduce yourself into change by teaming up with a friend who will enable you to be consistent. This aspect of getting fit—eating healthier—is no different. So, rather than pouring your energies and your resolve into one more diet, pour them into finding a partner, a friend which whom you can establish a consistent walking program or exercise routine.

As you treat your body better, through movement and activity, it will respond. It will begin to naturally crave exercise. Then, it will crave healthier foods. Not overnight, but in due time. Plus, with a friend along for the journey, it only takes one of you to take the lead in changing your eating ways—because the other will be close behind. Then, all the discipline that you've used to stay in your exercise routine can be transferred and applied toward helping you to make wiser food choices. When providing your body with regular activity becomes as routine for you as brushing your teeth, then you will be ready to see the concrete ways that a proper diet can serve you best.

The more fit you become, the more in tune with your body you will be. That will help you develop a stronger sense of what your body wants and when. You will *want* to treat your body better, in all ways, from food to exercise to sleep to relaxation. You will have all the incentive you need at that point to give it what it needs. You will have all the tools required to home in on a healthier way of life.

∼ Learning to Listen to Your Body ∼

At the stage when you are homing in on a healthy lifestyle, much of what you learn will be done through trial and error. You will need to test how your body responds to certain foods. This will depend on the intensity of your workouts, whether you are in training mode, or are simply in the groove of a regular routine.

When you are eating for performance or are training for a specific event, you will have the added structure of the goal to support a rigid eating program. During peak training, your body will demand that you feed it properly in order to reach your target. When you listen to your body, you will hear its request for hydration. How? You may experience headaches or flulike symptoms following an intense workout. While you may feel sick, you are actually dehydrated and your body is calling out for water. Or, during the day you may notice that your urine is dark yellow or even brownish; again your body is asking for water. After a late night of overeating, when you head out to train, you'll notice that you feel awful in comparison to the day when you ate small portions early on the night before. Could it be that smaller portions are better for you? You will need to listen long and hard to recognize the cues your body is sending you. Keep a journal of how you feel. And of course, chat with your friend.

While training for endurance events, you will be amazed at the intimate levels of detail you begin to share with one another about what your body is going through. You may have thought you knew each other well before, but that was just scratching the surface. What she discovers about her body's needs and reactions might help you, and vice versa.

When you're outside the parameters of a training goal, it's easy to backslide into more casual eating habits. As you'll find with your motivation, your eating habits will ebb and flow too. Once you have reached a specific goal, allow your body and mind time to rest. Use that time to take notes on your training experience, because in the process of reaching your training goal, you will have learned more and more about your body's needs. You will have learned so much, that it will be hard not to apply that insight to your normal day.

That's when you'll find yourself reading food labels and being shocked at the number of calories and the lack of nutrients contained in seven chips. You'll start to recognize that your body needs foods to keep it satisfied (and those seven chips are not going to cut it). You may start to move toward eating more fiber and whole grains, so you feel fuller longer. You'll be keenly aware of the types of foods that people eat that *don't* meet their body's needs and that don't satisfy. You'll start to invest time in researching the right foods for you and for your family. It's also when you've acquired the discipline and the wherewithal, that you notice how challenging it is to eat healthily in our society. Certainly, no social situations support it. Few restaurants do either (although all of them claim to do so in their ads and glossy menus). The good news is that by then, you will have become a person who eats to live, regardless of what everyone else around you is doing. The bad news is that while being fit and eating right can change your body—and your life—it's no guarantee that those changes will help you uncover that perfect "10" body that you think is lying buried underneath.

∽ Notes ∽

Write down how you feel after eating certain foods, before and after your workouts. Does pasta and shrimp the night before a workout help you feel full of energy and vigor? Does a half a banana before a dance class settle your stomach? Do you feel sluggish after you eat french fries? Also make note of how different foods make you feel throughout the day.

Capture the details about what works for you and what doesn't work for you. Then share your findings with your friend.

CHAPTER 10

THE BODY IN THE MIRROR

WHAT DO YOU SEE when you look in the mirror? It's hard not to focus on the faults, bumps, and imperfections. If you've struggled with your weight or have simply grown up in our society, you may dream of having the "perfect body." You may find yourself comparing every part of your figure against mythical, air-brushed standards—only to respond with self-hatred and disdain.

If your weight fluctuates at all, it can be a struggle to gain a true per-spective on how you look, because you may always see yourself heavy (or heavier than you really are) even when you're at your thinnest. As we get older, particularly as we head into our forties and beyond, and we begin to fight the aging process, that list of disliked pieces, parts, and places seems to triple. Each bulge becomes bulgier. Every dimple gets deeper. Gravity begins to take hold until our perkiest and firmest spots sag in despair. Even if you have the perfect body—and all other women wish they could be you—there's a good chance that you, too, want to change something about it. Learning to revere the body you've been blessed with *as you see it today,* rather than loathe it, is a tall order for most women. So, the question is: can "getting fit" alter what we see when we look in the mirror?

∼ Kim Looks in the Mirror ∼

As I was taking a shower last night, I stood and looked in the mirror. I hated what I saw. My butt droops in the back, just below the spot where I can see a trace of glut muscle. It looks to me as if I have two cheeks on each side, for a total of four butts. Two thick pads also seem to ring my waste, around the back part of my hips. They feel like shelves to place my hands on. My thighs are riddled with cellulite, particularly in the front and along the top part of my knee. And of course, I have maps of stretch marks on nearly every body part that's visible. As I stood there taking stock, all I could think of was, "Who do you think you are trying to write a book about fitness?!"

And then I reminded myself as I do several times a day that *being fit is not the same thing* as achieving the perfect body. One is attainable. The other may not be (depending upon your genes, your history, your body type, and how you've treated yourself in the past). Yes, it's frustrating to me that I can work out as hard and as often as I do and still be ashamed to put on a bathing suit. I hate that I'm comfortable only when wearing shorts that come just above my knee.

So why bother? Why be fit? Why exercise regularly, if it won't bring the one thing I've always wanted? Because being fit has brought me so much more than I ever imagined, more than I ever considered wanting. It's worth the concession. But it does take a concerted effort to remind myself of what my body is and what it can do, rather than to focus on what it is not.

At rest, my heart beats slow and steady. Yet when asked to work hard, it becomes mighty and strong. My legs, though they may jiggle in spots, are sturdy, as they carry me mile after mile after mile in our quest to run the marathon. My lungs respond in kind with vigor and stamina. My muscles and tendons constantly strive to deliver strength, stability, and power. My mind is clear, focused, confident, and driven. It doesn't shy away from challenge, obstacles, or quandaries. It knows how to dig down deep to find the courage to continue, even when it wants to quit. With ongoing challenges and being pushed to its limits, my body continues to respond, always becoming firmer, trimmer, slighter, stronger. My soul is satisfied, knowing what it needs to feel fulfilled and how it can reach out to others to connect. I feel as if I've become a well-oiled machine, with all systems working together efficiently and effectively, in peak condition.

I'll take all that I've discovered and achieved through fitness in lieu of having the perfect body. Even though I have to keep reminding myself that being fit is not the same as having the perfect body, I'll take being fit any day.

∽ Kris Looks in the Mirror ∽

As I stood on a raised platform, a doctor who specializes in veins was looking at the spider veins on my legs. As he carefully studied my legs, he stated that my legs looked "pretty good for my age." He agreed he could make some improvements, but he also offered some advice: be careful of seeking perfection; you will still have some marks remaining on your legs. A few weeks since the consult, his words and advice have continued to resonate in my ears. Today, I spend more time looking in the mirror than ever before. Is this because my appearance has changed so much that I am trying to establish a new visual for myself? Absolutely! Or, is it an attempt to realize that even with all the hard work and time spent exercising my body I still have so much room for improvement? Sadly, yes to this too.

Scrutinizing myself in the mirror is a relatively new habit for me. Even during college, when I first began to put on some extra pounds, I didn't spend much time obsessing about what I looked like in the mirror. Instead, as my clothes began to feel snug I turned to exercise to halt the mounting pounds. At the time, I wasn't the only one to gain weight. Most of my friends did too. College seemed to have that affect on us. However, my closest friend reacted to her weight gain by sticking her finger down her throat every time she overate. Clearly, my approach was a wiser, healthier one. But now, many, many years later, I realize that I only used exercise as a quick fix, a Band-Aid of sorts. Once the problem was remedied, I quit the exercise routine and seemed unwilling to make physical activity a priority or a regular part of life. That turned out to be a dangerous and foolish choice.

And it was quite a shift from life before college, when daily physical activity fit naturally into my life. Looking back, I wonder if the reason college was more difficult than high school was partly the result of my sporadic approach to activity. Moreover, I can't help but think that all of those years spent mired in health problems could have been reduced had I been more in tune with my body and confident enough to question the doctors.

Today I know that regular physical activity leaves you feeling energized. I know that the more you push yourself physically, the stronger you will feel mentally. I also know that the body constantly talks to you, providing you with ongoing information on what it needs—from the amount of rest required to which types of foods to eat to what activities to pursue to when to seek medical attention. Add to that the fact that your soul is also sending signals about what it needs to feel nourished and fulfilled, as well as what leaves it (and you) feeling drained and unhappy.

Yet armed with all that I know about what exercise and physical activity can deliver to my life—all of which is far beyond mere weight control—I still look in the mirror and find all my flaws. It's hard in today's world not to desire perfection or to at least want to improve your aging appearance. No longer do I see the shiny hair, fresh eyes, and dewy skin of the past. Even when people say, "You look great at your age," that doesn't really make me feel better.

The contradiction is that I do feel better about *what* my body can do, more than at any other time in my life. I can do "boy-style" push-ups. I can run mile after mile after mile without feeling winded or fatigued. If I can't currently do something, I no longer have any fear about trying a new skill. Marathon. Triathlon. Yoga. Pilates. Tennis. Time is now my only obstacle. Not only have I gained the confidence to pursue a variety of challenging athletic skills, I have the confidence to switch careers, to cowrite a book on fitness, and to colead and assist others in their pursuit of fitness.

So, maybe the image in the bathroom mirror causes my mouth to turn downward a bit, but all the while the mirror to my soul is smiling.

∿ Wishful Thinking ∿

So, yes, in a nutshell, getting fit can alter what you see in the mirror. It can, within reason, enable you to change your physique and the shape of your figure. More important, it can transform how you feel about yourself when you look in the mirror. You may never like the way that lump of fat sags over your kneecap. You may never get it to go away. Yet you may build a long list of things that you *do* love about yourself—from how your biceps bulge as you lift your grocery bags to how you can race bikes with your teenage son and laugh aloud as you beat him on the long stretch to how calm and centered you feel each evening. As your list of loves grows, your list of hates will shrink. Then, as you look in the mirror, you'll not only see what stands before you, you'll see yourself more practically, pragmatically, and wholly. You'll stop beating yourself up and begin to appreciate all that your body is and all that it can do.

So where does that process begin? It begins by taking two critical steps. You must:

- challenge yourself physically,
- learn to look at the positives and to think positively, rather than to focus on the negatives.

Let's explore these further.

Challenge Yourself

If you have already started walking with your friend, you might already understand how overcoming physical challenges can lead to greater confidence. One reason is that physical challenges are also mental challenges. In fact, some physical challenges seem to be all about enduring the mental challenge. Can you continue even as your mind begs you to quit? When you challenge yourself in this way—and do not give up—you will eventually see fitness gains. But, you will *instantly* see gains in confidence and self-assurance.

The sensation of saying, "Wow, I did it!" is a powerful one. The pride that wells up inside is uncontainable. Experiencing that time and time again will have a dramatic effect on your mind, your body, your soul. Your perception—the inner thoughts you hold about your body—will begin to shift. When this happens, it is as if all of the puzzle pieces—mind, body, and soul—fall into place. You will see yourself in a new and different light.

This phenomenon varies from what you'll experience with challenges that are solely mental ones. Those challenges—such as solving a complex work-related problem—can also deliver deep feelings of power and self-confidence. But they don't do anything to shift your perception of your body and its capabilities. You might feel clever, smart, and resourceful, but you'll probably still hate what you see in the mirror.

Challenging yourself physically can be done at any and every fitness level. For example, when establishing a walking program, the first set of physical challenges you will encounter may involve overcoming that sensation of being winded, as well as adjusting to having tired legs and sore muscles. However, each day that you continue on your walking program, you will notice that your body responds by getting stronger. You will feel less winded as you walk. Your leg muscles will become accustomed to the activity and will no longer feel sore and tired. This will last until you decide to challenge yourself again by increasing the frequency, the intensity (pace), or the distance of your walks. Again, in short order, your body will respond. This ongoing cycle forms the foundation for "how to" improve your *physical* fitness.

At each stage, as your body responds and adapts to the latest set of challenges, your mind responds as well. It begins to feel more confident, more in control, more capable. With each new challenge, it too will rise to the occasion (if you let it!). Soon, your body and mind will work in tandem to tackle the physical challenges you throw at them.

Running concurrent to this is the fact that your regular doses of friendship are feeding your soul. Its growing sense of fulfillment will help to ease your mind and calm your body. With a satisfied soul, fewer worries will plague you. Your mind will feel less drained. Without as many problems gnawing at you, you'll feel it within your body too. Maybe your heart will race less and less. Your stomach will no longer churn and knot. You will feel quieter inside and more at peace.

But the key is to maintain the *entire* cycle. First and foremost, you don't want to abandon your partnership and put your soul at risk of not getting what it needs. You also don't want to give up or to quit when faced with a physical challenge (since that can lead to poor self-esteem and a lack of confidence). So, you must *be sure that the challenge is appropriate for your fitness level.* Don't try to run five miles when a steady jog/walk for a single mile is a sufficient challenge. Set yourself up to succeed, rather than to fail. The more successes you experience, the greater your sense of achievement. You'll feel empowered. Then you will start to realize that if you can do this, you can take on a host of other challenges, physical and otherwise. You will begin to see that together, your mind and your body can accomplish anything! That's one of the major milestones for being able to more naturally appreciate—and revere—the body that you see in the mirror.

Think Positive Thoughts

The concept of learning to think positively, rather than negatively can apply to a variety of situations and moments. In terms of challenging yourself physically, you will need to learn to think positive thoughts and to literally coach yourself through various experiences. That's because our minds are powerful and tricky. As quickly as your mind can dream a dream, it will dream up reasons why and how you can't actually achieve that dream. Learning to fight the negative thoughts is one of the greatest skills that exercise can teach you.

With each challenge, you will notice a myriad of negative thoughts that come flooding to mind. Fighting those negative thoughts requires you to simply replace them with positive ones. At first, your mind and body may scream: *this is too hard . . . it hurts . . . I can't breathe . . . I feel sick . . . I'm uncomfortable . . . I can't do this!*

Push back those thoughts and replace them with equally powerful, positive thoughts.

- So, the next time you hear yourself say: "I'm dreading this." Stop and tell yourself instead: "This is going to be a good workout," or, "This struggle will make me stronger," or, simply, "I can do this."
- If you hear yourself say: "I suck at this," say to yourself instead: "Hey, at least I'm here, that's more than most people can say!" or, "I'm doing far more now that I was doing last week, two weeks ago, or last month!" or, "Look how far I've come already!"
- If you increase the intensity of your exercise, and your mind starts to rebel with: "This is brutal; I can't go on," tell yourself: "I'm going to settle into a rhythm," "I'm stronger than I realize," or simply, "Relax. I'm going to be fine."

Any and all of these positive comments can help. Pick one that feels natural for you to say. Then practice saying it repeatedly, even before your workout, so that you commit it to memory. It may sound silly and feel awkward at first, saying something positive to yourself, but it will go a long way toward changing how you feel during your workouts (and at other times throughout your days).

You and your partner can also help each other practice positive thinking. You can say aloud to one another: "We're almost there," or, "We're doing great, let's keep it up," or, "Look at how much stronger we are now!" Take every opportunity to pat yourselves on the back—before, during, and after your workouts—to keep your progress in perspective!

Learning to think positively and to be kind to yourself can extend outside your workouts. In fact, we often assault ourselves with negative thoughts throughout our days. "I hate my thighs . . . I am so fat . . . My gut is huge . . . I'm an idiot . . . I wish I was funnier . . . God, I look so ugly in this dress." As long as these types of thoughts echo in your head, you will never be satisfied with how you look or feel about yourself in general—even if you do happen to achieve your idea of "perfection."

Again, like you would during a workout, replace your negative chatter with something kind and empowering, such as: "I'm capable and smart . . . I'm in the process of becoming the best I can be . . . I am fitter, stronger, more powerful today than I was yesterday . . . I feel better than I have in years . . . I have a lot to offer . . . I'm on my way . . . I'm moving closer to my goals . . . I'm proud of myself . . . I may not have perfect (thighs), but I do have great-looking (arms)." And remember what Naomi Judd once said, "Your body hears everything your mind says."

∾ Changing What You Can, ∾ Accepting What You Can't

Combating the struggle of body image and thinking positively also requires understanding what you can change and accepting what you cannot. In practical terms, that means knowing that through exercise and proper eating, you can lose weight and transform your figure. You can also, of course, improve your health. However, depending upon your body type, your health history, and your age, you may never be able to make all of the changes on your wish list. Plus, it may not even be clear to you today what is changeable and what is not. You may simply find that you look back one day and realize that what was once an issue for you, no longer is.

And that's how it works. Because of your body's ability to constantly adapt to challenges, being fit becomes a lifelong pursuit, a never-ending journey that will allow you to look back over your accomplishments and ahead toward new goals. You won't arrive somewhere and then be done. Just as you reach one milestone, you'll find yourself waiting to discover another one worth pursuing. Better still, with each milestone the prospect of not exercising—of giving up your routine—will become more and more unthinkable. So be patient with yourself. If you spent a lifetime not exercising, it may take time for your body to respond. In the meantime, stop looking for some elusive finish line. Learn to live in the moment, enjoying the journey, and praising your body for what it is and what it can do here and now.

∾ **Notes** ∾

Write down some of the negative thoughts you frequently tell yourself, during workouts or throughout your day. For each one, come up with two to three *positive thoughts* to replace them.

_____

_____

_____

_____

_____

_____

_____

_____

∼ **Notes** ∼

Write down the one or two things you realize you may never be able to change about your body. Next, write down as many aspects about your body that you *have* been able to change during your fitness journey. *Or,* if you are new to the fitness journey, brainstorm to come up with a list of the changes you'd like to eventually see.

CHAPTER 11

LISTEN TO THE WHISPERS

I F YOU PROGRESS along the fitness journey linking the phases of a satisfied soul, a strong body, and confident mind, you will reach a time when the doors of opportunity burst open for you. Anything will seem possible. Moreover, you will be keenly aware of what you want and need to live a rich and fulfilling life.

If you take a moment to look back at our time line, you can see exactly where we started to reach this point. You can see the acceleration of accomplishments, as we explored new areas, launched new endeavors, and tackled new challenges. All of that arose from being strong, confident, empowered, and most important, in tune with the whispers emanating from our souls.

～ Kim Looks Back ～

In 1994, exactly ten years ago, I was at home folding laundry. I was pregnant with my second son and had a toddler roaming my house. I clicked on the *Oprah Winfrey Show*. She was training for her first-ever marathon, at the age of forty. They showed a film clip of her on a training run, in a rural part of Illinois, running alongside a cornfield. She was laughing, almost deliriously, at something she found funny. The entire show profiled her training program.

As I watched, I thought to myself, "That's amazing. I wish I could do that." Then in the shadow of that same sentence, I thought, "I could never do that." I vacillated between being envious (because I knew that she too had weight, self-esteem, and self-control issues) and being convinced that there was no way in the world, that I would ever be able to do anything remotely close to that physical feat. Twenty-six point two miles? Running? I hated running! I hated exercise. Period. But wow, Oprah's doing it. That was something.

It's now 2004. I am forty-one years old and have just completed my very first marathon. And I love running. Plus, not only do I love to exercise, I'm building my entire life—apart from what centers around my husband and children—around the pursuit of fitness.

Sometimes on long runs, I have something akin to a spiritual experience. I feel healed. And as I'm running I'm overcome with emotion. Occasionally, when I reach a certain distance—a stretch goal perhaps—I get misty-eyed and choked up, moved to tears that I am accomplishing my goal. Many times, an old song will play on my sport radio—something from days long ago, like a tune from Led Zeppelin or the Allman Brothers, that would have been the soundtrack behind my smoking, drinking, and driving fast—and I can't believe it's me here, plodding along, step after step, mile after mile.

I also can't believe that the focused, disciplined, and determined me that I've become was once so fragile that I was overwhelmed and reduced to tears when given a potted orchid as a gift from my husband. My, how things have changed. Hard to imagine those two women are in fact one in the same. Impossible to imagine that ever happening today. It feels good to be treating my body and my self so much better. It feels good to be healthy and strong, in every respect. It feels good to think: this is who I was meant to be.

I believe the day I watched the Oprah show that the faint glimmer of envy I felt was in fact a whisper. A whisper of buried passions lying deep within my soul. Back then, I wasn't tuned in to whispers. It was reflexive to say, "I couldn't do that." Or even stronger, "I could *never* do that!" as soon as something piqued my interest. Followed by, "I'm too fat. I'm too old. I'm too out of shape. That's not my thing. I'm not talented enough. I'm not smart enough. I'm not athletic enough. I'm not good enough at that kind of stuff."

Those words, those phrases, no longer cross my mind. Anything seems possible. Granted, I may not want to do something. I have no desire to sky dive. Yet I know I could, if I wanted to. Certainly it would take proper training and instruction. But I have the courage. I have the wherewithal. I go for it, when I want it. That's a far cry from thinking that you can't do something (even if, deep down inside you want to). That's also a far cry from being the fragile person who melted into tears when given a potted plant.

Today, if I hear a whisper it's usually greeted with the question, "What do I need to do in order to be able to do that?" or, "When is the right time for me to do that?"

Now it's all about having a plan. It's all about timing. After all, "where there's a will, there's a way." Feeling fit, balanced, and centered has given me all the will in the world, to find a way.

∼ Kris Looks Back ∼

When I was young I pursued many interests—gymnastics, dance, baby-sitting, vocal lessons, and reading. I moved freely from one activity to the other, satisfying all of my heart's whims and desires. At the age of sixteen, when I became treasurer of the Junior Achievement Club, I discovered I had an interest in the financial aspects of running a business. That spark, for many years, shaped my career.

Is it possible to know what you want to do for the rest of your life, at the tender age of sixteen? Perhaps. Unfortunately, I never really asked myself those questions. Instead, I followed my life's plan somewhat blindly, often being motivated by fear and by guilt. So, as I entered adulthood, I never considered that the goals I was pursuing might have changed from when I was younger. Or, worse, that there might be undiscovered passions and goals lying dormant and going unfulfilled.

It was important to me to have a career and to be independent, largely because of my parents' divorce. When they split up, the increased costs of maintaining separate households was a challenge. My mom had to return to work. Because she lacked professional training, she felt it best that she also return to college. I watched the struggles of my mother: managing three children, earning her degree, making her way back into the workforce, and balancing our finances. She didn't want me to face the same dilemma. Neither did I. I was terrified of being in that same, vulnerable position some day. So my determination to go to college and find a financially stable career drove many of my decisions. It never occurred to me to look beyond my interest in business finance and to explore other, unrelated professional arenas or fields.

Then, years later, when I was home on maternity leave caring for my son, I wondered how I could leave him. At the same time, I was fearful of leaving my career. What if something happened to my husband and I had to support my son? I compromised by going back to work part-time. Still, each time I left him I had a knot in my stomach. Was that the by-product of not listening to a whisper?

As time passed and I endured my five-year struggle with doctors and infertility issues, the realization sank in that I would never nurse another baby, never rock a baby to sleep again, or feel a little one hold round my leg to stay close. Worse, I felt a strong sense of guilt at not being able to provide a little brother or sister for my son. I feared he'd be lonely. Plus, I felt tremendous guilt over depriving my husband of the chance to have another child. To compensate, I threw myself into the role of supermom, snatching up volunteer jobs right and left, as I juggled my son's schedule.

It was during our walks when I first found the time to reflect on the course of my life. I realized that some of my career goals existed to stave off my childhood fears. Yes, it had been important for me to learn that I could be independent, a breadwinner, and resourceful. But once I'd learned that and the fears I'd held since childhood were gone, shouldn't I have earned the freedom to venture down some different paths? And yes, I found it fulfilling to work hard at being a wife and mother, and to volunteer for the community. But I also found myself feeling as if I were stretched too thin.

I began to realize that being motivated by fear or guilt—especially over things I could not change—had led me astray. I had been chasing goals that I no longer understood. My goals, formed long ago, were not reflective of the woman, the "me," that I'd become. And while I loved the involvement of volunteering for the schools and the community, the guilt had motivated me to go a bit overboard in my commitments.

The walking and talking with Kim gave me the chance to pull my head up, to look around, and to ask myself some hard questions. I realized that when I listened to my heart's whispers, it was beneficial to my soul. Was there a way to do both? Did meeting my family's needs mean I could only be selfless? Was it selfish to try to pursue some of my own interests and passions? I started to look for ways to marry the two—to weave the pursuit of my whispers into my life and to balance them with my current responsibilities. I slowly began to reshape how I spent my days.

Today, after many years on my soul-searching fitness journey, I am refocused. I am now pursing a completely different career, one that leaves me energized rather than drained. And since it's hard to hide my enthusiasm, my son sees how a life, a family, a career, can be framed by the things that bring you joy, the things you love to do. I hope it will encourage him to follow his dreams and to listen to his whispers. I know that many people no longer recognize the person I have become. But the fact is they're simply—finally after all this time—-seeing the true person I was meant to be.

∿ What Whispers Do You Hear? ∿

Whispers often come when we're in the company of others. Perhaps a friend is telling you a story about how she is learning to sail a boat. The thought crosses your mind that you might like to learn to sail too. In an instant though, your mind discounts the idea and the thought vanishes.

Take some time over the next few days to complete these journal exercises. First, try to remember the times when someone mentioned a pursuit, a talent, a passion, or an accomplishment that piqued your interest, but that you quickly dismissed (for whatever reason) as something that you could never do. Write them down in the space below.

Tracking your whispers can be done at any time during your journey, even if you're just starting out. Because while you may not feel the confidence or gumption to pursue them today, in time you will if you continue along on your fitness path.

∽ **Notes** ∽

Take time today to notice whenever someone mentions a pursuit, a talent, a passion, or an accomplishment that seems to resonate with you. Before you dismiss it, write it down here.

\
\
\
\
\
\
\
\
\
\
\
\
\
\
\

∽ **Notes** ∽

Make a list of the types of comments that your negative voice makes to discount your whispers. For example, "Oh you're too fat to ever run a marathon," or, "You don't have any artistic talent to pursue a hobby like painting." Then, think of some positive thoughts that can combat the negative ones.

Whisper:

_____

Negative Voice:

_____

Positive Thought to Replace It:

_____

Whisper:

_____

Negative Voice:

_____

Positive Thought to Replace It:

_____

∽ **Notes** ∽

Now, look back at your list of whispers. List the top two that you would like to pursue or accomplish most.

1. Getting Fit

_____

2.

_____

3.

_____

You'll notice that we've filled in the first whisper for you: *getting fit.* Clearly, we're assuming that you are reading this page in the early stages of your journey and that you bought this book because a voice is telling you that's what you want. It's a goal worth pursuing. If you achieve it, we can very nearly promise that all of your other whispers—no matter how long your list—will also be within reach. But your first step is to find the will to follow the principles in this book, find a friend, then find a way to succeed at getting fit together. Remember: *if we can do it, you can do it.* And once you do, everything else will follow.

Appendix A:
Our Favorite Clothing and Gear

When we first started going to the gym we wore leggings and long, baggy T-shirts. We'd pick out our workout clothes on Sunday night or Monday morning and they'd last *all week long*. That's because we hardly ever broke a sweat. They were in perfectly good enough shape to wear during our next day's workout and the next day and the next day. That's how mild and moderate our workouts were. That's quite a contrast to where we are today, when we get chilled during the ten-minute drive home because our clothes are drenched. But as we've moved along our fitness path we've also veered off on some fashion adventures.

∽ Kris Looks Back ∽

Both our clothing and workouts have evolved over time and at the same pace. When we first began our morning walks, I could wear the same T-shirt and shorts for a week. When we moved to the gym and began weight training, I began to wear tank tops and shorts (which required washing every other workout). Once we started Don's kickboxing class, I discovered those clothes no longer worked. So I had to give up one of my favorite outfits—black gym shorts with an oversized muscle shirt. The shirt was huge to hide all my bumps and lumps, but it was exactly what I felt most comfortable in at the time. As I started to sweat more in his class, my discomfort with my appearance became secondary to the discomfort I felt wearing a weighted-down cotton T-shirt.

I needed shirts that did not retain sweat and cling to my body. I needed pants or shorts that did not ride up my bottom ever time I did a squat. So, we began searching and testing out various clothing options. One bra that we found by Under Armour was so comfortable it quickly became a favorite. Because it retained so much sweat, I discovered it was best worn alone or as a wicking layer under a wind breaker on a cool day running outside. Unfortunately, I learned that lesson the hard way! There I was in Don's class sweating profusely. The longer the class ran, the more I noticed something funny in the mirrors. From a distance, it was hard to make out. It looked as if there was something growing on my chest. As I sweated more and more, two perfectly round, large, circles began to appear on my tank top around my breasts. I continued to watch them grow darker and larger. I kept wondering how I was going to handle the situation and I just knew that Don had noticed—I only hoped he'd spare me the comments and ridicule. As soon as the class finished, I spun around, grabbed my cover shirt, and slid it over my head as I slipped out of the club.

Clearly, what works for one activity does not always work for another. What works for one level of intensity may not transfer to another level. The search for the right clothing goes on. All of which explains why the fitness clothes that once occupied a small corner in my drawer now take up an entire dresser.

∼ Kim Looks Back ∼

Several months after we started following a fairly rigorous training program in preparation for the half marathon, I was on the lacrosse field on the first hot day of the spring season. As I watched my boys practice, I noticed a nasty, rank smell. "Wow," I thought to myself. "Someone's got some bad BO!"

That someone was me.

As I stood there on the field, I could almost watch a pit stain growing beneath my arms as sweat rolled down my sides. Drips were starting to run down the canal where my cleavage should be. My back was drenched. I could actually feel beads cascading down the back of my legs. It was as if my body had transformed into a spigot.

My cotton tank clung to me and I worried that from the back view, my shorts had a huge wet stain on my rear from sitting in my chair. But the soggy look didn't bother me nearly as bad as the smell. I pinched my arms at my sides tightly, hoping no breeze would come along and carry the stench elsewhere.

"What is going on?" I wondered. I'd never in my life, ever been a heavy sweater. And I'd certainly never smelled like one.

Over the next several weeks, Kris and I both noticed that we were sweating more. At the drop of a hat, anywhere, any time. With all of the training, our bodies had begun to operate like well-oiled machines. At the slightest sign of heat, they started to work to cool us off; instantly purging any toxins that might be within and striving to keep our body temperatures regulated. Of course, being cool and comfortable did nothing for our general appearance!

We started to try new deodorants to rectify the problem. We searched high and low. Some left ugly, permanent white stains on our clothes. Others didn't seem to do much to fix the odor. One day, Kris mentioned the problem to a good friend who was a personal trainer. She laughed. Yes, she said, that happens when you get really fit. She recommended an "extreme" deodorant that worked well for her. It was a deodorant and antiperspirant combination. We gave it a try and it worked wonders.

For years, I thought that most of the features and benefits that were touted by fitness products were mere marketing hype and had little to do with substantive claims. I was dead wrong. Many products have been developed in the true interest of solving a problem or making the fitness pursuit more comfortable and enjoyable.

The trainer's recommendations made us realize that there are a host of products, accessories, and clothing on the market designed to meet specific fitness needs. We became more inclined to try them, buying clothing that had "wicking" fabrics and testing out antichafing products. I started wearing clothes made of special fabrics, not just when I worked out, but around town and throughout my days. Although I always looked like I was going to or coming from the gym, I felt incredibly comfortable. They kept me warm in winter and cooler, drier in summer. Gone were the pit stains. Then, I started to branch out and try some of the items besides clothing that were on the market. And I'm happy to report that nearly all the gear I've invested in—from water belts to GU—have helped make a difference in some way, shape, or form.

This appendix outlines some of our favorite clothing and gear—from the basics you can use on day one of your walking program to more performance-oriented gear that will help when your workouts get hard. We have grouped our recommendations by type of exercise and have included a general section featuring items that can benefit you regardless of your sport or activity.

∼ What Not to Wear ∼

What you decide to wear during your time at the gym, while walking, or during any workout can make or break your experience. Here are some basic tips for those first early days:

- Don't settle for wearing some old pair of aerobics shoes you found in the back of your closet from the days you used to take step aerobics classes. Instead, buy yourself a decent pair of walking, running, or cross-training shoes. (Running shoes can be used for walking, but walking shoes should not be used for running. If you intend on doing any jogging or aerobics, consider getting a good pair of shoes that are appropriate for the activity you want to try).
- Don't wear cotton socks. Buy yourself some cushioned athletic socks, preferably with a wicking fabric. Again, for walking or any other type of aerobic activity, good socks are key. They'll prevent blisters and make your feet more comfortable (and less stinky!).
- Don't wear your everyday bra. Invest in a quality athletic bra, preferably one with wicking fabric. Regardless of the size of your chest or the intensity of your workout, a comfortable and supportive athletic bra can make a big difference in how you feel when you're moving, bending, stretching, jogging, walking, or jumping. One of our favorite manufacturers is Under Armour, because their fabric is lightweight and silky, and it magically wicks away moisture so you don't get chilled or chafed.
- Don't worry too much about how you look. Your priority is to be comfortable during your workouts. You don't want to be tugging or pulling at your clothes, or feeling pinched or bound in any way. Find some attractive outfits in which you can move, bend, jump, and twist.
- Don't assume cotton is king. There are so many high-tech fabrics on the market that will keep you comfortable and dry during your workouts, that you don't need to settle for an old cotton T-shirt and your old 80s leggings and scrunch socks. Go

out and treat yourself to a workout outfit or two (on sale of course!) You'll be glad you did.

∾ General Clothing and Gear ∾

Sports Bras

A sports bra should provide adequate support, fit tightly but not be too binding, and keep moisture away from your body. They are best paired with a tank top or a loose-fitting top made from a wicking fabric. This is better than pairing it with a cotton shirt, because the T-shirt will absorb the sweat that the bra wicks away—therefore defeating the purpose of the bra's wicking features. If you are uncomfortable wearing the bra on its own, there are models that combine a sports bra and a tank. To our knowledge, no sports bra will adequately hide nipples.

When you are purchasing a sports bra for the first time, it's best to try on the various models in a store. Once you find a design you like and know the exact size, then you can purchase them online.

Our Favorite Sports Bras

- Under Armour. We love Under Armour products because of the feel of the fabric and the seamless designs. They carry a variety of styles. The sports bra tank design is a good option if you don't want your midsection exposed, although it does fit snuggly against the body.

  One of the downsides of Under Armour, is that their fabrics are so good at soaking up moisture, that the wetness often starts to bleed onto any shirt that you wear over it. Therefore, sometimes the Under Armour bras are best worn alone, without another shirt over them—especially if you're doing a highly intense workout or run. However, the sports bra tank helps address this issue because it eliminates the need for a cover shirt and hides the belly at the same time. (www.underarmour.com).
- Nike. Its line includes a wide selection of built-in bra tanks that are mesh. They allow for ventilation and are a looser, lighter fit around the midsection (www.nike.com).

- Moving Comfort. This company has an extensive line of clothing made specifically for women athletes (www.movingcomfort.com).

Socks

Blisters are a common running and walking injury. Be sure you find socks that fit properly and will keep moisture away from your feet. Look for socks made of synthetic materials such as CoolMax, Dri Fit, Dryline, polypropylene, and Intera.

Different thicknesses are available: light, medium, or heavyweight. Try the various styles to determine your favorite.

Our Favorite Socks

- Ultimax Ironman Triathlon
- DeFeet Air-E-Ator Cush
- Thorlo running socks

General Gear

Even if you have a large gym bag and will need to shower and change at the gym, carry a smaller bag or satchel with you to your classes or onto the gym floor itself. A small shoulder bag can hold your water, ID card, a jump rope, towel, tampons, extra shirt, tissues, and cycling shoes. Be sure to keep it all organized and ready to go so that you're not searching for it each morning or afternoon.

∾ Running Gear ∾

Shoes

You can walk in a running shoe, but you cannot run in a walking shoe! To purchase a quality running shoe from salespeople who understand the sport, go to a store that specializes in selling running shoes. They will outfit you correctly.

Some dos and don'ts to consider while you're at the store:

- Do not rush.
- Do not be shy.

- Do talk about how many miles you will run in a week, or whether you're training for a race or particular distance, or if you're a beginner;
- Do talk about how you may roll your feet when you run—outward or inward (supination or pronation).
- Do ask them to watch you run if you do not know whether you roll inward or outward.
- Do talk about any feet or leg pains you may be experiencing.
- Do take your old shoes along so they can be examined for signs of supination or pronation.
- Do ask them to make note of the particular model you purchase within their computer system as well as the size, so that you have a record of your shoe (in the future, you may forget which model you bought and you may want to buy another pair).
- Do consider purchasing a half size larger, to allow your feet to swell or expand during exercise.
- Do look for models with a roomy-sized toe box, to allow your toes to move.
- Do try the shoe on with the type of sock you intend to wear.

You may want to purchase two pairs of running shoes at the same time, even if they are the same model. This can lengthen the life of your shoe and give you an alternate pair to use. It can also prevent a particular shoe from causing irritations and, if they are different models, allow you to work slightly different muscle groups. Just remember to order or purchase your shoes well in advance. For example, if you place an online shoe order and your shipment is delayed by any length of time (because of a backorder), you risk having to run in shoes that are breaking down. While this may not be an issue for the runner who is logging two to three miles at a time, it is a huge issue for someone who is running ten to fifteen miles at a time.

Other Running Accessories

- Wear identification on your shoes. Purchase a Velcro ID medal to attach to shoes. If you don't have an identification tag, at least slip a business card in your pocket.

- Run with a water belt. Staying hydrated is important, regardless of the temperature outside. But certainly, it's extremely critical when it's hot out. There are a host of different options for staying hydrated, from belts that carry several small bottles to camel-pack hydration systems. The one that's right for you will largely depend on your personal preference.
Most single-bottle styles are designed for the water to be carried in the nook of your back. However, if you don't like the sensation of that weight pulling on your stomach while you run, turn the belt around so that the water bottle sits in front, making sure it's cinched tightly so it doesn't bounce.
- When running in hot weather, wear a terry cloth wrist band. This will come in handy to keep the salty sweat out of your eyes and to dry your face. A sweatband can also be doused with cold water to help keep you cool.
- Use sunscreen and lip balm. Remember your shoulders, your nose, and the backs of your knees.
- Wear a baseball-style cap/hat or visor. Hats and visors, made of wicking materials can help keep sweat out of your eyes. They're also great for keeping a sweaty mop of hair out of your face and off of your neck.
- Wear sunglasses. Obviously, sunglasses help shield the glare, so you can be more comfortable. But they also keep gnats and bugs out of your eyes and protect them from particles of dust.
- Use antichafing products to prevent blisters and raw skin. If you start to have a problem with chafing or would like to prevent blisters, consider using petroleum jelly or a special antichafing product that you can purchase at running specialty stores that glides or rolls on wherever you need it.

Our Favorite Sunglasses, Hats, and Visors

- Maui Jim Titanium Sport sunglasses (flexible and lightweight)
- Nike Dri Fit sun visor (also available in a baseball-cap style)

～ Outfits for Warm Weather–When ～ It's Fifty Degrees or Warmer

To outfit the rest of your body, you must consider the weather as well as your personal preferences and comfort. But when it's warm outside, it's a good idea to wear as little as possible. Whether it's warm or cold out, *don't wear cotton.* When it's hot, cotton absorbs sweat and moisture, and will weigh you down. When it's cold, cotton absorbs sweat and chills you, particularly when you're transitioning from running to walking, either during a workout or a cooldown.

Shorts

Consider loose shorts with built-in panties. Find garments made of synthetic materials that keep the moisture away from your body and do not rub or chafe while you are running. We have found that it is difficult to find running shorts that are long enough for our comfort level that also have pockets. Pockets are necessary to carry tissue, car key, cell phone, and a business card (for identification's sake).

Our Favorite Shorts

These manufacturers usually offer a model or two that we like, though their products do change regularly:

- In Sport. We like the length of these shorts and the feel of the material. The company also has a model with pockets, although it does not have built-in panties (www.insport.com).
- Road Runner Sports. Love the material, length, and built-in panties but do not have pockets (www.roadrunnersports.com).
- Moving Comfort. This company has a longer-style short that is lightweight, has pockets, and is extremely comfortable (www.movingcomfort.com).

If panties are not built in the short, consider purchasing a pair that are made with CoolMax or Dri Fit.

Long-Sleeve Shirts

When the temperature is only fifty degrees it may be a bit cold to start out in a bra top or tank. Wear a loose-fitting, lightweight, long-sleeve (noncotton) shirt that you can take off and tie around your waist once you warm up.

Our Favorite Shirts

- Nike Dri Fit (short sleeve and long sleeve)
- Under Armour (short sleeve and long sleeve, loose or tight fit)
- Road Runner Sports (long-sleeve shirts)

～ When It's Cold Outside—Less ～ than Fifty Degrees

Layering will be key to staying comfortable when it's cold. If you step outside prior to your run on a cold day and are comfortable in the elements, then you are overdressed. You should be slightly chilled. As you warm up on your run, your body temperature will rise. As it does, the chill will go away and you'll be comfortable. Again, *do not wear cotton.* When it's cold, cotton will also absorb sweat and chill you.

- Layer 1 is the clothing next to the skin. Its role is to keep moisture away from the body. All clothing you have selected for your warm-day runs can be used for your first layer. You may also choose to wear moisture-wicking panties versus shorts to avoid bunching.
- Layer 2 is the insulating layer. You want to move the moisture to the outer layer but you also want to trap warm air.
- The outer layer protects you from wind, rain, and snow. Look for jackets made with microfiber, Gore-Tex, Polartec, or ClimaFit. Make sure the material is breathable, so that sweat can escape. Avoid styles that are bulky and prohibit your movement. Make sure you have pockets that zip shut. You will get hot on cool days and want to shed your hat and gloves, so you will need a pocket to store them. Also a jacket that is relatively lightweight is easier to tie around your waist if you get hot. Finally, look for jackets

that feature vents along the back shoulder blades or near the arms, which can be zipped open, in case you want to cool off.

Leggings

As with jackets, look for pants made with microfiber, Gore-Tex, Polartec, or ClimaFit. Look for zippered pants pockets as well. We prefer to wear styles that are closer fitting, so that they don't bunch or twist around our legs. Be wary of some types of windpants that do not have lining. On cold days, unlined windpants can either cause a chill, or if you start to sweat, cling to your legs. Also consider a pant that fits tightly around the ankle to avoid cold air entering through your leg. Some pants have a zipper at the bottom, to allow you to open up a vent if you get too hot and want some cool air to circulate.

Our Favorite Leggings

- Hind
- Under Armour Cold Gear
- Any CoolMax or Dri Fit tights

Hat and Gloves

Choose a hat and gloves that are thin but designed to insulate and keep you warm. You may also consider an ear band, just to cover your ears if that's more comfortable for you.

When it's chilly but not too cold, wear glove liners rather than heavier gloves. They will keep your hands from getting too cold but are lightweight and breathable.

～ Aerobics and Cross Training ～

Shoes

Perhaps the item that will mean the most to you during any aerobics or cross training activity will be the shoes that you wear. A host of shoes are specifically designed for aerobics and for cross training. Or, you can consider wearing a good running shoe. Whichever you choose, you should consider having more than one pair to workout in. You don't want to be wearing the same pair of shoes every day for all your activities. Varying the model and the pair will help give your feet a rest and prolong the life of each pair of shoes.

Clothing

Comfort is king when it comes to clothing that you wear in a class. This is especially important if you are going to be facing a mirror for the entire time. Make sure you're okay with seeing yourself in that outfit for a prolonged period of time. But realize, you're going to make mistakes. Search for a tight supporting bra, preferably one that will hide your nipples (if you find one let us know). Patterned bras seem to work best for this issue.

How much you sweat during the class will influence how comfortable you are in your clothes. If you have two big sweat-based bull's-eyes on your breasts once the class if over, you'll be miserable. Always grab a towel before class to help you through those awkward moments (it's easy to clutch a towel to your chest, discreetly, as you grab your gear.) Throwing an extra shirt in your gym bag helps too (as long as the bag is in the class with you.) You can quickly throw it on and get out if you need to. Again, cotton T-shirts won't cut it in a high-intensity class.

Being comfortable also translates to how you're feeling that particular day. Some days, you may feel plump, pudgy, like you want to hide. That's a good day for a loose-fitting tank and leggings. Other days, you may feel thin, strong, and on top of the world. That day you may feel brave enough to sport some cute shorts and only a sports bra. Your comfort level with what you wear and how you feel about yourself will fluctuate from day to day. All you need is to make sure you have the clothing options you need to support how you feel on any given day. (This may mean not only purchasing enough but also making sure you keep up with the laundry so that there's always something clean to match your mood.)

∼ Cycling and Spinning Classes ∼

If you get hooked on a cycle class, we highly recommend investing in cycling shoes that clip into the bike pedals. More so than anything, the shoes make a difference in the cycling experience. They give you a smoother pedal rotation and the ability to pull up with your quads.

Bike Shorts versus Leggings versus Regular Shorts

Whether or not you choose bike shorts or leggings or regular shorts to cycle in depends upon your own personal preference. If you want more cushion on your tush, consider bike shorts and a gel seat combination (you can take the gel seat on and off for each class). If you will be looking at yourself in a mirror the entire time you pedal, think about what you need to wear in order to be comfortable with what you see. Also, consider the creep factor. During cycling classes, many shorter-style leggings can creep up your leg. Decide how long they need to be so they are not distracting and annoying. While much depends on personal preference, we don't recommend wearing shorts in a cycle class or pants that are loose around your ankles and legs because they can flop around and get caught in the bike chain. Ditto for the laces on your shoes. If you hear the clicking sound of your laces hitting the gear guard, make sure they're secure enough to not get caught in the chain.

An entire industry has sprung up around performance gear and clothing. Once you get hooked on the options, you'll want to explore the many catalogs, Web sites, and stores that cater to this market. Best of all, you'll never run out of great gift ideas for your friend at birthdays and holidays. In fact, you may be the only person who repeatedly has the ability to buy her exactly what she wants and needs.

Our Favorite Catalogs and Web Sites:

- Athleta (www.athleta.com)
- Title Nine Sports (www.title9sports.com)
- Road Runner Sports (www.roadrunnersports.com)

Appendix B:
Posture and Activity Tips and Techniques

Within the past year, in our pursuit to become certified personal trainers through the National Academy of Sports Medicine, we have learned tips, techniques, and cues regarding proper posture and form for many common exercises. We've included some in this appendix to provide you with a quick reference guide and concrete guidance designed to keep you safe and to avoid injury.

~ Posture ~

When you begin any exercise, and even throughout your day, here is how your body should be positioned for optimum alignment and posture:

- Stand with your feet shoulder distance apart.
- Feet should be pointing straight ahead.
- Pelvis should be in neutral. (To find neutral, stick your butt out as far as it will go, then tuck it under as far as it will go, then find the position right in the middle.)
- Draw in your abs. (Pretend as if you are pulling in your stomach to zipper a tight pair of jeans. You should draw your belly button in toward your spine.)
- Tighten your gluts. (To see if they're engaged, take your thumb and give yourself a little poke in the butt to see if they're tight.)
- Your shoulders should be back and down. (Not hunched around your ears. Try to pull them back and down, as if tucking them into your back pocket.)
- Your head should be in alignment with your ears, right above your shoulders.

- Tuck your chin slightly, as if you were holding an apple beneath it.
- Practice this proper form while at the grocery store, in your kitchen, and throughout each day.

∼ A Walking Program ∼

This walking program is outlined in the beginning of the book, but we've included it here as well for quick reference. It will provide you with a structured approach to help you establish a walking program in a more methodical way.

Week 1: Start with a ten- to fifteen-minute walk at an easy pace. You should be able to carry on a comfortable conversation, without feeling winded. Walk three to five days the first week. Again, building your routine is your primary goal, so consistency is important.

Week 2: Add three to five minutes of walking a day, up to twenty minutes.

Week 3: Add three to five minutes a day, up to twenty-five minutes

Week 4: Add three to five minutes a day, up to thirty minutes.

Once you are up to thirty minutes a day, walking three to five times a week, you can begin to pick up your pace a bit each day. This will allow you to cover more distance within the same amount of time and increase the challenge.

∼ Tips ∼

1. If you find walking for the suggested amount of time to be too difficult, cut back on the number of minutes, then repeat that schedule for another week or two, until you are able to progress comfortably.
2. Increase the time you spend walking each week before you increase your walking speed.

3. Be a good partner. If your companion feels aches and pains, slow down the pace and don't be in a rush to "achieve" a certain milestone.
4. As you walk, be aware of your posture. Think of lengthening your body with your head up, ears positioned over your shoulders, and your eyes forward. Hold your shoulders down and back, yet relaxed. Imagine tucking your shoulder blades into your back pocket. Tighten your abs and your gluts, and engage your muscles as you stride.
5. Your "rest" days are as important as your activity days.
6. Be sure to drink plenty of water before, during, and after your walk.
7. You should begin every walk with a slow warm-up. This means a slow-paced walk for three minutes or so. You can also add some gentle stretching after your warm-up and before the main portion of your walk.
8. Remember on your walks to enjoy the moments. Check out the homes' landscaping. Notice the critters on your block. Enjoy the scent of the dew on the grass. Listen to crackles of the leaves and crunching of twigs beneath your feet. Best of all, listen to the giggles and squeals of laughter coming from you and your friend.

∼ Basic Static Stretches ∼

Standing Hip Flexor/Calf Stretch

Many people suffer from both tight calves and hip flexors, especially women who frequently wear high heels. This stretch addresses both areas.

- Begin in your proper stance.
- Hinge back from your hip as if you are beginning to sit down on the toilet. (Make sure you don't just stick your butt out, hinge at your hip, and let your torso follow, keeping it in a straight line).
- Take one full step back with your right leg.
- Plant your heel firmly on the ground (your front leg should be slightly bent).

- Tuck your pelvis under.
- Gently lean forward, until you can lean no more without sacrificing form.
- Hold for twenty seconds and then switch legs.

You may or may not "feel" this stretch. It is a subtle sensation in your calf and in your hip flexor.

Ninety-Degree Hip Flexor/Quad Stretch

Whether walking, cycling, or running, this stretch can help lengthen your quad muscles and open up your hip flexors, so you can experience full range of motion.

- Lower yourself to the floor so that your right leg is bent at a ninety-degree angle. Your foot should be directly below your knee in a straight line.
- Your left leg should be bent so that your knee is on the floor. Be sure that your calf extends straight back, with your toes resting on the floor.
- Tighten your abs and your gluts.
- Tuck your pelvis under and hold that stretch for twenty seconds.
- Then switch sides.

IT Band Stretch

This is a great stretch for runners, because it lengthens the long and strong IT (iliotibial) band that runs down the outside of the leg. Runners often complain of pain associated with the IT band.

- Lie down in the supine position (on your back, with a neutral pelvis. Your back will have a natural arch, but it shouldn't be pronounced).
- Cross your right leg over your left and rest your outside right ankle on your left knee.
- Slowly pull your left knee in to your chest as far as it will go without hurting.

- You can hold your left leg beneath your knee to stabilize yourself or to increase the stretch.
- Hold for twenty seconds then switch legs.

Neck Stretch

This stretch can ease the tension in your shoulder and neck area, and is particularly helpful if you spend a fair amount of time at the computer.

- Begin in your proper stance.
- Take your arms and hold them down by your sides, flex your right hand, and extend your palm down to the floor.
- Tilt your head to the side so that your left ear lowers toward your left shoulder.
- Hold for ten seconds.
- Maintaining the same general position, raise your head slightly and look left over your shoulder and down toward the floor.
- Hold for ten seconds.
- Then take your head and move it at a forty-degree angle and look across your body to the upper right corner of the sky or ceiling.
- Hold for ten seconds.
- Switch sides.

Pectoral Stretch

This stretch can help open up your chest area and reduce the roundness that you might find in your shoulders, which often results from sitting hunched over for hours at a desk.

- Begin in your proper stance.
- Hold each arm at a ninety-degree angle in front of you with elbows bent at shoulder height.
- Draw in your abs to anchor your core.
- Slowly move your arms back, keeping them at a ninety-degree angle, until they are in line with your sides.
- Pinch your shoulder blades back, tuck them in your back pocket (do not hunch them up around your ears).

∽ Cycle/Spinning Classes ∽

If you're new to a cycling class, be sure to arrive early to check out the equipment and to make sure it is adjusted for your height. Ask the instructor to help you adjust the seat. The seat should be at roughly the same level or height as your hip bone. When adjusting the handle bars, higher is better, initially for comfort. As you get more experienced you can lower them into more of a racing position. It's a personal preference regarding the distance between your handle bars and your seat, but you don't want to be too stretched out. Also, ask the instructor where the emergency stop button is on the bike. This allows you to instantly stop the pedals, in case your foot flies out. This prevents the pedals from continuing to rotate at high speeds and smacking you in the calf (ouch!).

As you're pedaling, keep your foot flat and don't lead with your toes. Instead, pull up with your quads when you go around. Keep your stomach in so your back stays flat, to work your ab muscles. Your arms shouldn't be flexed outward; keep your elbows tucked in at your sides so you don't put too much weight on your wrists. Keep your shoulders down and relaxed. Focus on your form rather than on intensity, especially at first, because cycling with improper form won't help you get the best workout. It'll become more natural after a while. And you'll be at less risk for injury. Cycling shoes can help you maintain proper form, because you can pull your legs up and around during the revolution (rather than pushing down with the opposite foot to propel the turn.)

If you start to love cycling classes, nothing will work as well to tighten your butt and your quad muscles and to help you build shapely legs. However, fair warning: your legs will *increase* in size simply from the added muscle mass. Be prepared to have your shape change and to feel as if your pants may be getting tighter, especially around your upper thigh area. It's certainly a good thing, but if you've struggled with body image and are tied to how certain clothes feel on you, it will take a shift in perspective to realize that your tighter clothes are a good sign, not a bad one!

∾ Muscle-Sculpting Classes ∾

Muscle-sculpting classes may introduce you to:

- Hand weights (dumbbells) and bars. Many sculpting classes rely on exercises that can be done with dumbbells and bars to work your biceps, triceps, shoulders, and back. Be careful in any class not to try to keep up with what everyone else is doing. It's far better and more effective to do five repetitions correctly, than to do one hundred incorrectly! Even if the instructor is going on and on and on with biceps curls, if you can no longer do one with proper form, then you *need to stop* and put your weight down or decrease the weight and resume proper form. Improper form is the leading cause of injury. So, instead, take a rest. Then resume again, if or when you can. Work hard to engage or activate the proper muscles. If you're doing biceps curls, you shouldn't be swaying forward and backward in order to lift the weight. Keep your trunk stable and strong, by tightening your abs. Do controlled movements, rather than hoisting the weights up with momentum. In time, your abilities will increase and you'll be able to do more and more. If you're not sure about what you should be focusing on in terms of proper form, ask the instructor (who should be shouting out cues along the way throughout the class). If you're too shy to ask, then have your friend ask.
- Squats. The benefit of squats is that they can ease back pain, strengthen your gluts and quads, and help define muscles in your legs. Again, they must be done correctly. Proper form for a squat includes having your hips shoulder distance apart, with your feet pointing straight ahead. Allow yourself to lower to a squat as if you're getting ready to sit on a toilet, pushing your butt slightly back toward the wall behind you. Don't let your knees extend past your toes. Don't adjust your head and neck so you're looking up. Instead, your head and neck should be at a slight natural angle, in line with your spine so that you are slightly gazing at the floor in front of you. Lower yourself only as far as you can go maintaining proper position. If your chest

starts to sink toward the floor and you're leaning forward, you've gone too far. As you get stronger, you will be able to sink lower. Push up through your heel, tightening your gluts to propel you to a standing position.

- Push-ups. Doing a proper push-up is perhaps one of the most challenging exercises we know. But when done correctly it delivers more concrete results, quicker than any other single exercise we've found. It will shape your triceps, your biceps, your back, your shoulders, as well as your butt and hamstrings! Again, if done correctly. In a proper push-up, your body should be straight as a plank. In the "up" position, your head should not fall forward. Keep your chin slightly tucked, as you pull your head back to be in line with your spine. Don't let your shoulders roll forward. Your legs should be fully extended and you should be on your toes. Tighten your abs, your gluts, your hamstrings, your calves. Your arms should be along your sides, with your elbows beside your ribcage. Slowly lower yourself, maintaining your plank position. Do *not* let your head fall forward to meet the floor before your chest does. Do *not* keep your butt in the air as you only lower your chest to the floor. Again, think strong, stiff, board. Lower yourself, then push yourself back up, again maintaining your position. Doing even one correctly may be all that you can do. That's okay. Build from there. When you're in a class, remember these cues. If you're working on push-ups outside of a class setting, your friend can spot and cue you to make sure you have proper form.
- Stability Balls. These balls are a great way to improve your core strength. Just be careful as you get on and off them or as you change positions, because they can easily pop out from beneath you and send you crashing to the floor. If you and your friend are working on them outside of a class, hold the balls for each other as you get on and off. When you're on a stability ball, your primary goal is to engage your core (the muscles in your abdomen and back) to keep you stable. Try not to rely solely on your quads and calves, though certainly they can assist your core.

∾ Running ∾

One of the safest ways to work into a running program is to use a run/walk approach. Jeff Galloway, a running guru and the biggest proponent of "walk breaks" has written several books and developed a host of materials to help people get started. His advice is great for beginning and advanced runners alike. (He also has a Web site: www.jeffgalloway.com.)

Here are some general principles common among running programs and trainers, including the concept of walk breaks, that will help keep you injury free and feeling strong as you kick off a running program:

- As you run, maintain a tall posture. Look up ahead, rather than down at your feet (especially when you're tired). Keep your chest high, your arms and hands relaxed (not clenched in a fist.) Don't hunch your shoulders up. Keep your arms down, with your hands swinging at belly button level (not at chest height). Try to stay relaxed as you run.
- Work up to your distance gradually. Never increase your distance by more than 10 percent in any week. If you are starting out on a running program, you need to develop a baseline from which to build your mileage. During your first week, each time you run, you should only go for roughly ten minutes or so, and certainly no more than a mile. Even if you've been walking many miles for many months, you should *not* kick off a running program by simply trying to run that same distance. You may however, run for ten minutes, then continue to walk for the rest of the distance. This can help ease any sore muscles that occur from running. If you find it difficult to run for the entire ten minutes, then you should run for one minute, walk for one minute, alternating run/walk breaks.

  Follow this routine three days a week only. Each week, simply add another minute or two to your running time, until you build up to twenty minutes. At that point, you have a solid base that you can begin to add half-mile increments to *one* run day each week, until you reach your desired distance. The other two days however, should still be twenty-minute runs (with walk breaks if necessary). Ideally you should stay at an increased distance for two weeks or more, before you increase by another half mile.

- Incorporate stretching in your routine, as well as a proper warm-up and cooldown. Stretching is a critical component to healthy running. Yoga and Pilates classes can serve double duty as stretching routines.
- Let your body rest. Running is hard on the body. Therefore, your rest days are as important as your run days. Rest days can consist of cross training or any non-weight-bearing exercise. The goal, however, is to give your feet and your legs a rest from the pounding.

When you run, take it slow and steady rather than fast and sporadic. Go for a sense of control at your pace, your speed, your level. Don't compete with others and feel compelled to run at a pace that's not comfortable for you. Also, do your best to control your breathing so that you're not gasping. Use your walk breaks to recover.

Appendix C:
A Journal for Your Journey

Hopefully you have chosen a friend, decided on your plan together, and are ready to begin your journey together. Review your notes from the exercises at the end of chapters 1 and 2. Write a quick summary here:

Chosen friend: _____

Our plan is to:

_____

_____

(Recap where you'll meet, what days and times you'll meet, and what you'll do together. If you've decided to kick off a walking program, review the tips in chapter 2. You may also want to refer to chapter 3 for ideas on how to connect and what to chat about during your time together.)

On the following pages you'll find a journal to help you and your friend throughout your journey. There are three sections, one for each phase of your journey. Phase I is to help you chronicle how you and your friend *nurture your souls*. Phase II will help you track how you *challenge your bodies*. And Phase III will help you as you *cultivate the power of your minds*. Some pages feature prompts and questions to guide the chats you and your friend have. Other pages are blank. You can make copies of them if you wish, before you journal your thoughts and feelings. We've also included a basic fitness log which you can reproduce and keep in a binder or folder.

∽ Why Keep a Journal? ∽

Keeping a journal is a powerful process that will enable you to delve deeper into your thoughts, perceptions, and challenges. The journal will chronicle your growth and change. It will help you shape your dreams and vision. Lastly, keeping a journal allows you to look back and remember key moments, inspirations, and ideas.

Make several copies of the blank journal pages, then take a few minutes each day to capture your thoughts. Use the journal pages for as many months or years as you need to, in order to capture your journey together. On each anniversary of the day your journey began, treat yourselves to a healthy lunch and look back over what you both have written in your journal pages. Praise yourselves for your accomplishments and rejoice in how far you've come *together*.

∽ How to Journal ∽

If you are not in the habit of keeping a journal, you will likely feel uncomfortable and awkward in the beginning as you struggle to capture and put down your thoughts. These simple guidelines may help:

1. **Don't censor what you write.** No one else will read this journal, unless you choose to let them. So don't worry about how your words sound, how they're written, or whether they are spelled correctly. Simply write down what pops into your mind. Your journal entries should be stream of conscious activities, where your mind is free to wander and roam unencumbered.

2. **There is no wrong answer.** Nothing you write down will ever be "wrong". So don't be afraid to write exactly what's on your mind. Even when your thoughts are painful, negative, hateful, and embarrassing, be brave. Write them down

3. **Give yourself at least 10 minutes each day to complete your journal activity.** Most of the exercises have been designed so they can be completed in a short amount of time. One suggestion is to complete your journal activity in the morning. That will give you the rest of the day to mull over the more thought-provoking questions even further.

4. **Don't be afraid to revisit an activity page.** After you've completed an activity, you may find that more thoughts rush to mind. Or your thoughts become more clear and refined. Go ahead and revisit that activity page and write down your additional thoughts and capture that clarity. You can use the back of each page if you need more room to write.

∽ Phase I Nurture Your Souls ∽

Begin your journey right here. After your walk (or workout) today with your friend, return to this page and write down your thoughts and feelings.

How do you feel right this minute?

I just returned from our walk or our workout together and I feel . . .

_____

_____

_____

_____

_____

_____

_____

_____

_____

_____

_____

_____

_____

_____

_____

_____

What did you talk about? What did you laugh about?

_____

_____

_____

_____

_____

_____

_____

_____

_____

_____

_____

_____

_____

_____

_____

_____

_____

_____

_____

_____

_____

_____

_____

_____

_____

_____

_____

Make several copies of this page, then each day take a few minutes to capture your thoughts and memories of your journey together.

Write down what you talked about, what you learned, what made you laugh, and how you felt when you were done.

_____

_____

_____

_____

_____

_____

_____

_____

_____

_____

_____

_____

_____

_____

_____

_____

_____

_____

_____

_____

_____

_____

～ Phase II Challenge Your Bodies ～

If you have spent time nurturing your souls and are ready to increase your intensity and to challenge your body more, you may also be ready for a different type of journal—one that will track your goals and your progress more specifically.

Create a Training Plan

If you're looking for ideas of how best to challenge your body, refer to your notes from the exercises in chapter 7 and to appendix B: Posture and Activity Tips and Techniques. Whenever you set a goal, be it to train for your first 5k race or to increase your upper body strength, you need a training plan. Below is a sample plan, followed by blank pages that you can complete yourselves. Make copies and put them to work for you. Work together to complete your training plans, so that they outline your goals and strategies clearly.

Sample Training Plan

> **Our goal is to . . .**
>
> *Build our upper body strength*
>
> ---
>
> **We want to meet our goal by (set a realistic date):**
>
> *We want to start to see an increase in strength and maybe some better muscle definition by March 16th, which is 8 weeks from today.*
>
> ---
>
> **Our plan is to. . .**
>
> *Attend one muscle sculpting class each week on Wednesdays at the Community Center, and then get together two additional times in our basements, for a 20 minute workout with some hand held weights.*
>
> ---
>
> **We will consult the following training experts or resources for our plan . . .**
>
> *Consult with a personal trainer for one hour, so she can devise a safe, effective plan for us to follow.*
>
> ---
>
> **We will meet . . . (location, time, days of the week, frequency)**
>
> *Wednesdays at the class at the Community Center for their 6:00 a.m .class; then Mondays and Fridays from 6:30 a.m. to 7:00 a.m., alternating homes each week.*
>
> ---
>
> **Potential obstacles we need to address include:**
>
> *If one of our husbands goes out of town on business and we can't meet in the early morning.*
>
> ---
>
> **Our plan for these challenges is to . . .**
>
> *Use Tuesdays and Thursdays as alternate days to get together, if Mondays and Fridays get derailed.*
>
> ---
>
> **We will track our progress by:**
>
> *Using a daily log to detail the weight lifted, number of reps and sets.*
>
> ---
>
> **We will be able to measure our results by:**
>
> *Being able to track whether or not we can do more sets and reps and/or increase the weights we use.*

Our Training Plan

Our goal is to . . .

We want to meet our goal by (set a realistic date):

Our plan is to. . .

We will consult the following training experts or resources for our plan . . .

We will meet . . . (location, time, days of the week, frequency)

Potential obstacles we need to address include:

Our plan for these challenges is to . . .

We will track our progress by:

We will be able to measure our results by:

Training Log, Week of: _____

Goal this week:

Ultimate Goal:

Date/Day	Activity	Distance/Time of Workout	How did you feel? (Comments)

∿ **Phase III Cultivate the Power** ∿ **of Your Minds**

If you have nurtured your souls and challenged your bodies, you may be ready to cultivate the power of your minds. Simply put, this means taking the discipline skills, the confidence, and the sense of resolve you've developed so far together and applying it to new and different areas of your lives.

You and your friend should work on these exercises together. Grab your pens, journals and a copy of our book and get ready to unleash the power within!

First, re-read the chapter on Whispers. If you haven't yet done so, jot down your list of Whispers and complete the exercises in that chapter. Once you're done, take a few minutes to list the things in life that you would like to do and to accomplish before you die. *Don't censor what you write.* Just scribble away, without thinking about how, when, or even why you would want to accomplish such challenges. Next, pick one from your list that you would like to improve or change *immediately* (assuming you've already accomplished the first one we wrote for you, which was to: *get fit.*)

Now answer these questions . . .

If you don't achieve these changes immediately what will that mean to you?

_____

_____

_____

If you *do achieve* these changes, what will that mean to you?

_____

_____

_____

Once you're done, map out your plan for how you will achieve your se-lected goal and how each of you will support the other.

∽ Our Powerful Minds Plan ∽

Make copies of this page so you can use the format again and again to tackle different goals, assess and track your progress. Each week, update the steps you will take and the ways you will measure your success.

My goal is to . . .

Deadline for reaching my goal (set a realistic date):

My friend's goal is to. . .

Her deadline is:

Three steps I can take over the next several weeks to move closer to my goal:

Three steps she can take to move closer to her goal:

The primary step I will take this week and next week will be to . . .

The primary step she will take this week and next week will be to . . .

I will support her by doing or saying the following . . .

She will support me by doing or saying the following . . .

I will be able to measure my success by:

She will be able to measure her success by:

Index

NOTES

NOTES

NOTES

NOTES

NOTES

NOTES

NOTES

NOTES

NOTES